# FIRST AID FOR THE®

# Radiology Clerkship

**LATHA G. STEAD, MD**

Chair, Division of Emergency Medicine Research
Professor of Emergency Medicine
Mayo Clinic College of Medicine, Rochester, Minnesota

**MATTHEW S. KAUFMAN, MD**

Fellow in Hematology
Long Island Jewish Medical Center, New Hyde Park, New York

**S. MATTHEW STEAD, MD, PhD**

Consultant, Department of Neurology
Mayo Clinic, Rochester, Minnesota

**ANJALI BHAGRA, MBBS, DMRD**

Postgraduate Diploma in Diagnostic Radiology
Department of Internal Medicine,
Mayo Clinic, Rochester, Minnesota

**NORA E. DAJANI, MD**

Resident in Radiology
Mayo Graduate School of Medicine
Mayo Clinic, Rochester, Minnesota

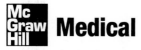 **Medical**

New York / Chicago / San Francisco / Lisbon / London / Madrid / Mexico City
Milan / New Delhi / San Juan / Seoul / Singapore / Sydney / Toronto

*The McGraw·Hill Companies*

First Aid for the® Radiology Clerkship

1 2 3 4 5 6 7 8 9 0 QPD/QPD 12 11 10 9 8

ISBN 978-0-07-138101-7
MHID 0-07-138101-5

---

### Notice

Medicine is an ever-changing science. As new research and clinical experience broaden our knowledge, changes in treatment and drug therapy are required. The authors and the publisher of this work have checked with sources believed to be reliable in their efforts to provide information that is complete and generally in accord with the standards accepted at the time of publication. However, in view of the possibility of human error or changes in medical sciences, neither the authors nor the publisher nor any other party who has been involved in the preparation or publication of this work warrants that the information contained herein is in every respect accurate or complete, and they disclaim all responsibility for any errors or omissions or for the results obtained from use of the information contained in this work. Readers are encouraged to confirm the information contained herein with other sources. For example and in particular, readers are advised to check the product information sheet included in the package of each drug they plan to administer to be certain that the information contained in this work is accurate and that changes have not been made in the recommended dose or in the contraindications for administration. This recommendation is of particular importance in connection with new or infrequently used drugs.

---

This book was set in Goudy by Rainbow Graphics.
The editor was Catherine A. Johnson.
The production supervisor was Catherine Saggese.
Project management was provided by Rainbow Graphics.
The index was prepared by Rainbow Graphics.
Quebecor World was the printer and binder.

This book is printed on acid-free paper.

**Library of Congress Cataloging-in-Publication Data**

Stead, Latha G.
    First aid fir the radiology clerkship / Latha G. Stead, S. Matthew Stead,
Matthew S. Kaufman.
        p. ; cm.
    Includes index.
    ISBN-13: 978-0-07-138101-7 (pbk.)
    ISBN-10: 0-07-138101-5 (pbk.)
    1. Radiology, Medical--Examinations, questions, etc. 2. Clinical
clerkship--Examinations, questions, etc. I. Stead, S. Matthew. II.
Kaufman, Matthew S. III. Title.
    [DNLM: 1. Radiology--Examination Questions. 2. Radiology--Handbooks.
3. Clinical Clerkship--Examination Questions. 4. Clinical
Clerkship--Handbooks. WN 18.2 S799f 2008]
    RC78.15.S86 2008
    616.07'572076--dc22
                                                        2008008579

# REVIEWERS

**M. FERNANDA BELLOLIO**
Escuela de Medicina Pontificia Universidad Catolica de Chile, Santiago, Chile
Research Fellow, Department of Emergency Medicine
Mayo Clinic College of Medicine, Rochester, Minnesota

**RAVNEET DHILLON**
Christian Medical College, India
Research Fellow, Department of Emergency Medicine
Mayo Clinic College of Medicine, Rochester, Minnesota

**BRUCE GARDNER**
Mayo Clinic College of Medicine, Rochester, Minnesota
Resident in Radiology, Mayo Graduate School of Medicine, Rochester, Minnesota

**ANN M. HOFF**
University of North Dakota School of Medicine and Health Sciences, Grand Forks, North Dakota
Resident in Emergency Medicine, Mayo Graduate School of Medicine, Rochester, Minnesota

**KUNAL JANI**
Mayo Clinic College of Medicine, Rochester, Minnesota
Resident in Radiology, Vanderbilt University, Nashville, Tennessee

**VEENA MANIVANNAN**
Kempegowda Institute of Medical Sciences, Bangalore, India
Research Fellow, Department of Emergency Medicine
Mayo Clinic College of Medicine, Rochester, Minnesota

**BALAVANI PALAMARI**
Gandhi Medical College, Hyderabad, India
Research Fellow, Department of Emergency Medicine
Mayo Clinic College of Medicine, Rochester, Minnesota

**BENJAMIN J. SANDEFUR**
Mayo Clinic College of Medicine, Rochester, Minnesota
Resident in Emergency Medicine, Harvard Affiliated Emergency Medicine Residency (HAEMR), Boston, Massachusetts

**KIM RYAN SCHUTTERLE**
University of Illinois at Urbana Champaign, Illinois
Resident in Emergency Medicine, Mayo Graduate School of Medicine, Rochester, Minnesota

**LUIS A. SERRANO**
Ponce School of Medicine, Ponce, Puerto Rico
Assistant Professor in Emergency Medicine
University of Puerto Rico School of Medicine, San Juan, Puerto Rico

**GITA THANARAJASINGAM**
Mayo Clinic College of Medicine, Rochester, Minnesota
Resident in Internal Medicine, Brigham and Women's Hospital, Boston, Massachusetts

**ABHIGNA VEDULA**
Rochester Community and Technical College
Undergraduate Student

# CONTENTS

# INTRODUCTION

This clinical study aid was designed in the tradition of the *First Aid* series of books. It is formatted in the same way as the other books in the series. You will find that rather than simply preparing you for success on the clerkship exam, this resource will also help guide you in the clinical diagnosis and treatment of many of the problems seen by radiologists, physicians, and trainees across several specialties.

The content of the book is based on the objectives for medical students laid out by the National Medical Student Curriculum in Radiology which may be viewed at: http://www.aur.org/amser/AMSER_national_curriculum.html. "Must see" images are incorporated into the chapters based on anatomy. There is also a practical section on "lines and tubes" that will come in handy for ward rounds in other clerkships.

The content of the text is organized in the format similar to other texts in the *First Aid* series. Topics are listed by bold headings, and the "meat" of the topic provides essential information. The outside margins contain mnemonics, diagrams, summary or warning statements and tips. Tips are denoted by  .

# HOW TO CONTRIBUTE

To continue to produce a high-yield review source for the radiology clerkship, you are invited to submit any suggestions or correction. Please send us your suggestions for:

- New facts, mnemonics, diagrams, and illustrations
- Low-yield facts to remove

For each entry incorporated into the next edition, you will receive personal acknowledgment. Diagrams, tables, partial entries, updates, corrections, and study hints are also appreciated, and significant contributions will be compensated at the discretion of the authors. Also let us know about material in this edition that you feel is low yield and should be deleted. You are also welcome to send general comments and feedback, although due to the volume of e-mails, we may not be able to respond to each of these.

The **preferred way** to submit entries, suggestions, or corrections is via **electronic mail**. Please include name, address, school affiliation, phone number, and e-mail address (if different from the address of origin). If there are multiple entries, please consolidate into a single e-mail or file attachment. Please send submissions to:

**firstaidclerkships@gmail.com**

Otherwise, please send entries, neatly written or typed or on disk (Microsoft Word), to:

> Latha G. Stead, MD
> C/o Catherine A. Johnson
> Senior Editor
> McGraw-Hill Medical
> Two Penn Plaza, 23rd Floor
> New York, NY 10121

All entries become property of the authors and are subject to editing and reviewing. Please verify all data and spellings carefully. In the event that similar or duplicate entries are received, only the first entry received will be used. Include a reference to a standard textbook to facilitate verification of the fact. Please follow the style, punctuation, and format of this edition if possible.

## INTERNSHIP OPPORTUNITIES

The author team is pleased to offer part-time and full-time internships in medical education and publishing to motivated physicians. Internships may range from three months (e.g., a summer) up to a full year. Participants will have an opportunity to author, edit, and earn academic credit on a wide variety of projects, including the popular *First Aid* series. Writing/editing experience, familiarity with Microsoft Word, and Internet access are desired. For more information, e-mail a résumé or a short description of your experience along with a cover letter to **latha.stead@gmail.com.**

## NOTE TO CONTRIBUTORS

All entries become properties of the authors and are subject to review and edits. Please verify all data and spelling carefully. In the event that similar or duplicate entries are received, only the first entry received will be used. Include a reference to a standard textbook to facilitate verification of the fact. Please follow the style, punctuation, and format of this edition if possible.

# CONTRIBUTION FORM

Contributor Name: _____

School/Affiliation: _____

Address: _____

Telephone: _____

E-mail: _____

Topic:

Location:

Cause:

Image findings:

Notes, Diagrams, Tables, and Mnemonics:

Reference:

**You will receive personal acknowledgment and a $10 gift certificate for each entry that is used in future editions.**

# How to Succeed in the Radiology Clerkship

## ▶ WHAT TO EXPECT

Radiology is an exciting and multifaceted field. Diagnostic and interventional radiologists utilize the multiple imaging modalities to identify pathology and treat disease. Many recent innovations and advancements in technology have allowed radiologists to obtain increasingly higher resolution images of the human body. Along with this increase in resolution comes the increasing responsibility to identify and distinguish between details that were once indistinguishable. Advancements in computer technology now allow for advanced 3D reconstruction and 3D modeling, which can also help aid patient care. Radiology truly is at the forefront of merging patient care with science and technology. As a medical student doing a radiology clerkship, you will likely get to see and work with many of the imaging modalities listed below:

- Radiographs or plain films
- CT
- MRI
- PET and other nuclear medicine studies
- Vascular/interventional radiology
- Ultrasound
- Many other new and upcoming technologies

Radiology is also unique in that the most challenging patients in the hospital often pass through the department. The pace can vary tremendously within the department. At times, the attendings may be too busy to acknowledge you, while at others extensive teaching on one case is possible. It is essential to remain interested and attentive no matter what degree of attention you are paid.

Residents in radiology tend to be very willing to teach medical students. Try to follow one closely, and offer to look up pertinent patient information whenever possible; this way, the resident will be keen to teach on interesting cases.

Remain responsible for your safety. Ask the allied staff politely where to source lead aprons, thyroid collars, etc. and be prepared to wear them in a prompt fashion. Learn how the different snaps and buckles work beforehand to avoid delaying the attending during procedures.

## ▶ WHAT TO BRING

There is very little you will need to have on your person while rotating in the radiology department. A basic list of equipment to carry with you includes:

1. One or two black pens
2. Small notepad to track patients and record important teaching points
3. A basic radiology introductory text such as the one you are holding

## ▶ WHAT TO WEAR (HOW TO DRESS)

Radiology as a field has many subspecialties, and the dress code can vary drastically according to the specific subspecialty. It is in your best interest to find out prior to your first shift what you are expected to wear. If for some reason this is not possible, men should dress professionally, wearing a suit with any color shirt and tie. Women should also wear professional attire in the form of a suit or business skirt and blouse. It is generally better to be overdressed than underdressed as it is much easier to change into scrubs if they are needed than vice versa. It is generally a good idea not to wear scrubs unless specifically instructed to do so.

## ▶ WHAT TO DO (HOW TO BEHAVE)

There are a few things we can say about what makes a medical student look good and excel during the radiology clerkship. This rotation will be unlike any other you have taken thus far. The attendings and residents at most institutions are aware that there is very little teaching and exposure to radiology throughout medical school. What they are looking for is a keen, interested, and intelligent student. A good grasp of anatomy is helpful, as this understanding of anatomy is fundamental to identifying the radiologic presentation of disease.

A few general pointers:

- *Punctuality* is very important! Being early will enable you to know what studies need to be read on the day, what the patient list looks like, and also which interventional procedures are going to be carried out.
- Work with the technicians to further your knowledge. For example, ultrasound techs are specially trained to perform the US examination, and an introduction to this invaluable technique may be gained by interacting with them.
- Try to show interest no matter how difficult the information seems to you or how little attention is paid to you.
- Hand in hand with showing interest is the important feature of being affable. Often you will sit and read with one attending all day. Being nice and polite goes a long way in making the day shorter.
- Asking questions on unclear topics is often necessary for effective learning. However, it is important to realize that interrupting the attending on every study is not acceptable, as they have to balance the need to teach with the requirement that the day's workload is completed. Ask questions when they are not too busy; otherwise, write down your questions and ask them at a later time.
- One way to enhance your experience and help facilitate learning is to read over some of the basic principles and review the anatomy relevant to the specific areas you will working with (e.g., if you are scheduled to be working in mammography, review the anatomy of the breast and the principles behind breast imaging beforehand). This quick review will serve not only to allow you to converse intelligently with the attendings, but will also earn you many bonus "points" if you are able to identify the anatomy.

## ▶ WHAT NOT TO DO

- Be late
- Make up an answer to a question you might not know (just say you don't know)

- Look sloppy
- Seem uninterested
- Turn down the opportunity to do a procedure (even if you've done it before)

## ▶ WHAT TO READ

Most radiology departments will have a departmental library for the use of the residents and staff. Oftentimes, you will have time dedicated in the schedule for reading. Ask the rotation coordinator, secretaries, or librarians if you can check out books, or if you have to keep them in the library. Useful texts *besides* this book include:

> *Essentials of Chest Radiology*—Felson's
> *Radiology Secrets*
> *Squire's Radiology*

Other useful resources include:

> Institutional/departmental teaching files
> http://brighamrad.harvard.edu/education.html
> http://apdr.org/documents/online_resources.cfm

## ▶ THE EXAM

The last hoop you will need to jump through before finishing the clerkship will be the final exam if one is given. Many departments will not require an exam and evaluations are based solely on personal interactions and "at the lightbox" questioning. It is in your best interest to find out the policy at the institution where you will be completing your rotation.

## ▶ A WORD ABOUT RESIDENCIES

Radiology attendings, residency directors, and department chairpersons will be observing you as a potential resident. You are, in a sense, auditioning for a position in the match. Residents you may work with can be your allies and help you "look good" to the attendings and ultimately attain a residency position (if this is your goal).

You are generally expected to do a rotation in your home hospital's department (the one affiliated with your medical school). Outside of that, it is always a good idea to do a rotation in the hospital where you would most like to do your residency. Fall is the best season for this, as it is the beginning of interview season. You will most likely get an interview, barring any medical disasters you may precipitate or gross personality conflicts with the staff. Interviewing after your rotation usually is more of a formality since most of the attendings have already worked with you and know you (see the advantage?).

While on your radiology rotation, it is a good idea to know a thing or two about radiation effects and safety. The biologic effects due to excess x-ray irradiation are a result of the interaction of high energy x-rays with atoms in DNA and other molecules in the body. These high energy x-rays have enough kinetic energy to ionize electrons that can directly damage the DNA or produce free radicals that can also be deleterious to genetic material, and may result in cell death or mutation. Most diagnostic radiologic exams expose patients to relatively low levels of ionizing radiation and are relatively safe. Radiology workers, however, are exposed to the cumulative dose of all examinations they perform and are therefore at a much higher risk.

In general, when performing radiologic examinations only the minimum amount of radiation necessary to obtain adequate test results should be used, and the benefits of doing the examination should outweigh the risks of performing the exam. Being well informed about radiation safety precautions is an essential skill for any good student on a radiology clerkship, for the benefit of both you and your patients. Generally, whenever ionizing radiation is being used, as in the use of x-rays for radiographs, fluoroscopy, and computed tomography, and you are in the immediate vicinity, be aware and use available protection (e.g., lead vests, thyroid and gonad shields). Also, be aware that many interventional procedures are carried out utilizing ionizing radiation (i.e., CT guided biopsies, ablations, angiograms, etc). Ultrasound and MRI exams do not produce ionizing radiation.

Lower-dose examinations include plain films, like a basic chest radiograph (x-ray). Higher dose examinations include computed tomography (CT) scans and scans involving the use of contrast dyes such as barium or iodine. It is important that as medical providers we do the best we can to keep track of a patient's x-ray history and make informed decisions about whether or not to proceed with a scan, especially in cases where clinical suspicion is extremely low and a radiologic study may not be warranted.

Pregnancy is also an important consideration in deciding whether to proceed with certain radiologic studies. While most modern radiologic studies do not pose a serious risk to a developing fetus, there is a very small risk of causing serious illness or other complications. This risk varies widely with the type of examination being performed—for example, ultrasound exams have not been demonstrated to increase risk in pregnancy. Similarly, plain film radiographs at sites other than the abdomen (e.g., of the extremities, chest) do not expose the developing child directly to x-ray irradiation. Delivering greater amounts of radiation, the risks and benefits of CT during pregnancy must be strongly weighed and these examinations are done much less commonly in pregnant women. It is important to be aware of the potential consequences of radiologic studies on pregnant women and that most institutions have specific guidelines regarding performing such examinations.

The dose of radiation a patient is exposed to varies from patient to patient. This dose will depend on the size of the body part examined, the type of procedure, and the type of CT or other equipment and its operation. Generally, radiation exposure is calculated as the "effective dose." The effective dose is evaluated in units of millisieverts (abbreviated mSv; 1 mSv [used for CTs] =

5

1 mGy [used for x-rays].) Using the concept of effective dose allows comparison of the risk estimates associated with partial or whole-body radiation exposures. This quantity also incorporates the different radiation sensitivities of the various organs in the body. Below is a table excerpted from http://www.radiologyinfo.org that gives some comparisons of effective radiation doses between various common radiologic procedures.

| PROCEDURE | EFFECTIVE RADIATION DOSE | COMPARABLE TO NATURAL BACKGROUND RADIATION FOR |
|---|---|---|
| CT—Head | 2 mSv | 8 months |
| CT—Sinuses | 0.6 mSv | 2 months |
| CT—Spine | 10 mSv | 3 years |
| Cardiac CT for Calcium Scoring | 2 mSv | 8 months |
| CT—Chest | 8 mSv | 3 years |
| CXR | 0.1 mSv | 10 days |
| CT—Abdomen | 10 mSv | 3 years |
| Intravenous Pyelogram (IVP) | 1.6 mSv | 6 months |
| Radiography—Lower GI Tract | 4 mSv | 16 months |
| Radiography—Upper GI Tract | 2 mSv | 8 months |
| Voiding Cystourethrogram | 5–10 yr. old: 1.6 mSv | 6 months |
| | Infant: 0.8 mSv | 3 months |
| Bone Densitometry (DEXA) | 0.01 mSv | 1 day |
| Hysterosalpingography | 1 mSv | 4 months |
| Mammography | 0.7 mSv | 3 months |

OK, good luck . . . enjoy the book.

# SECTION II

# High-Yield Facts

# Neuroradiology

## ▶ IMAGING MODALITIES

There are four main imaging modalities used to evaluate the head (Fig. 1-1):

- Computed tomography (CT) without contrast
- CT with contrast
- Magnetic resonance imaging (MRI) of the head with IV contrast*
- MRI of the head without IV contrast*

## ▶ CT LANGUAGE

Increased whiteness on a CT scan is referred to as **hyperdense** or **high attenuation.** Causes of hyperdensities include:

- Calcification
- Acute hemorrhage
- Ossification
- Contrast

Increased darkness on a CT scan is referred to as **hypodense** or **low attenuation.** Causes of hypodensities include:

- Air
- Fat

Note that air appears darker than fat on a CT scan.

## ▶ CT WITHOUT CONTRAST

### When to Order

This is usually the first test performed in an emergency setting. It is excellent at identifying blood.

### Advantages

If patient is stable, there are relatively no contraindications for ordering this test. It is a fast exam that can be completed in seconds.

### Disadvantages

Due to bony artifact, it is difficult to visualize abnormalities in the posterior fossa and brain stem.

---

* MRI is beyond the scope of this book; this chapter will focus primarily on CT.

## When to Order

If no abnormality is seen without a contrast, then a scan with contrast could be ordered to see if there is identifiable pathology. Contrast will help identify tumor, abscess, arteriovenous (AV) malformation, and aneurysm.

## Advantages

If a lesion enhances with contrast, then the blood-brain barrier is compromised. This can be seen in tumors, abscesses, and arteriovenous malformation.

## Disadvantages

Contrast will obscure an acute bleed. Thus, in an emergency setting, it is important to obtain a CT without contrast first.

## ▶ HOW TO PRESENT A CT SCAN OF THE HEAD (FIG. 1-1)

- First, confirm the CT belongs to your patient.
- If possible, compare to a prior film.
- Then present in a systematic manner:
  - **Technique:** With or without IV contrast
  - **Acute finding:** Check for blood, which will be bright white on a noncontrast scan.
  - **Cisterns:** Check the four key cisterns for blood or effacement: mesencephalic, suprasellar (star shaped), quadrigeminal, and sylvian.
  - **Brain:** Check for symmetry, low/high attenuation, midline shift, loss of gray/white differentiation.
  - **Ventricles:** Check lateral, third, and fourth ventricles for blood, shift, or effacement.
  - **Bone:** Look for adjacent soft tissue swelling and underlying fracture.

*Sample CT Presentation*

"This is a noncontrast axial CT of Mr. Smith. There is an acute subdural hematoma along the left hemisphere, causing effacement of the cisterns, and left-to-right midline shift. There is associated soft tissue swelling. No evidence of an underlying fracture."

HIGH-YIELD FACTS

Neuroradiology

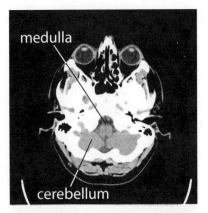

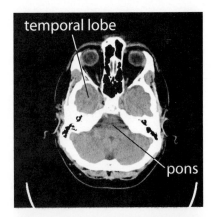

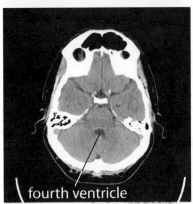

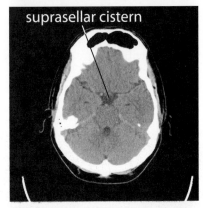

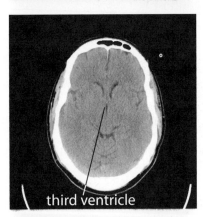

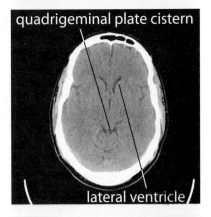

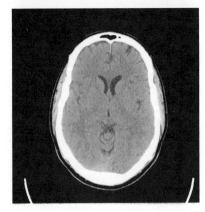

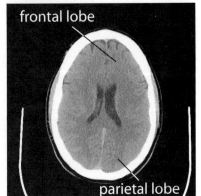

FIGURE 1-1. Normal CT anatomy.

## Skull Fracture

### CAUSE

Direct blunt trauma to the skull (Fig. 1-2).

### CT FINDINGS

Fractures can be classified as:

- **Linear:** Sharp lucent line with no depression of the fracture fragment(s).
- **Depressed:** Fracture fragments are depressed inward (Fig. 1-3).

Look for soft tissue swelling on the brain window setting to help identify an underlying fracture.

You may not see a skull fracture on axial images if it is in the same plane; you will need to look at the scout film to identify the fracture.

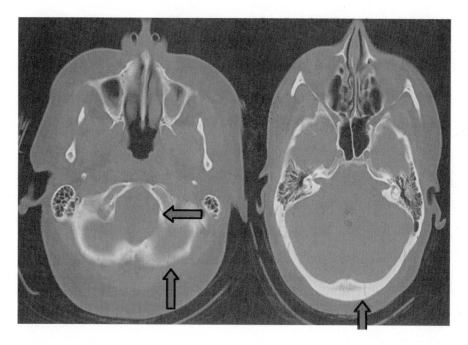

**FIGURE 1-2.** Axial CT bone windows show a nondisplaced communicated linear fracture of the left occipital bone extending into the lateral aspect of the foramen magnum.

HIGH-YIELD FACTS

Neuroradiology

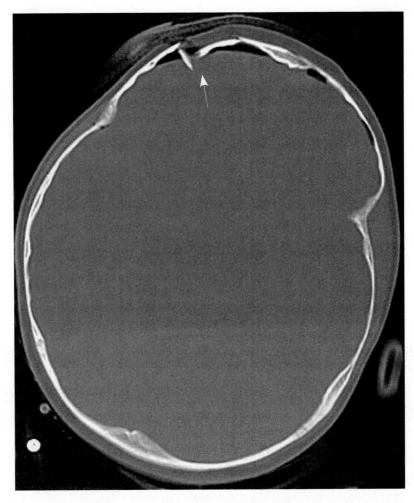

FIGURE 1-3. Axial CT bone scan demonstrating a depressed skull fracture (arrow).

## Subdural Hematoma (SDH) (Fig. 1-4)

### LOCATION

Ninety-five percent occur in frontoparietal regions.

### CAUSE

Most likely due to venous bleeding from tearing of the bridging veins.

### CT FINDINGS

- View in blood windows setting (width 250, level 40).
- Crescentic in shape
- Often extends into the interhemispheric suture and along tentorium
- Can cross suture lines, not midline
- Look for effacement of sulci.

*SDH Rule of Threes*
- Acute hematomas are crescentic in shape and hyperdense up to three days
- Subacute hematomas are isodense from 3 days to 3 weeks
- Chronic subdural hematomas are hypodense > 3 weeks

Suspect nonaccidental trauma in children with mixed-age SDHs.

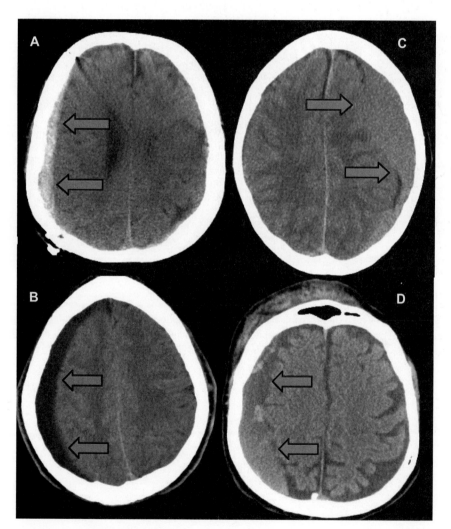

**FIGURE 1-4. Subdural hematoma.**

(A) Axial CT shows a hyperdense acute SDH along the left hemisphere. (B) Axial CT shows an isodense subacute SDH along the left hemisphere. (C) Axial CT shows a hypodense chronic SDH along the right hemisphere. (D) Axial CT shows an acute on chronic mixed SDH.

### Acute Epidural Hematoma (Fig. 1-5)

#### LOCATION

Seventy to seventy-five percent occur in temporoparietal region.

#### CAUSE

Most likely caused by laceration of the middle meningeal artery. In children it could be due to tearing of venous sinuses.

#### CT FINDINGS

- Usually associated with underlying fracture (85% to 95%)
- Does not cross suture lines but can cross the midline
- Biconvex shape
- "Swirl sign": Mixed areas of high and low attenuation is indicative of an acute bleed.

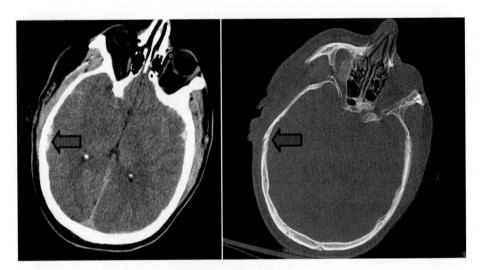

**FIGURE 1-5. Acute epidural hematoma.**

Axial CT shows a high-density extra-axial biconvex fluid collection along the right temporal parietal lobe (A); bone windows demonstrate an associated temporal bone fracture (B). Findings are all consistent with an acute epidural hematoma.

## Carbon Monoxide Poisoning (Fig. 1-6)

### LOCATION

Globus pallidus, cerebral and cerebellar white matter, sparing subcortical fibers

### CT FINDINGS

- Hallmark is symmetric, low-attenuation changes in the globus pallidus.
- May see on CT scan within 24 hours

**Carbon monoxide** is the number one cause of accidental poisoning deaths in the United States.

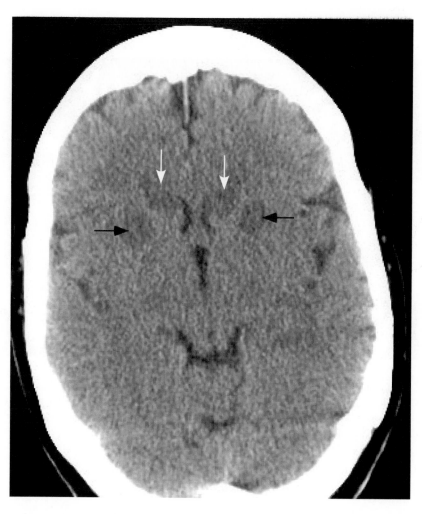

**FIGURE 1-6. Carbon monoxide (CO) poisoning.**

Note symmetric and low-attenuation changes within the caudate (white arrows) and putamen (black arrows), bilaterally due to anoxic event from CO poisoning.

### Subarachnoid Hemorrhage (SAH) (Fig. 1-7)

#### LOCATION

Occurs in the subarachnoid space

#### CAUSE

May be secondary to trauma or rupture of an aneurysm

#### CT FINDINGS

- Areas of hyperdensity within the cisterns and sulci
- Could produce posttraumatic communicating hydrocephalus

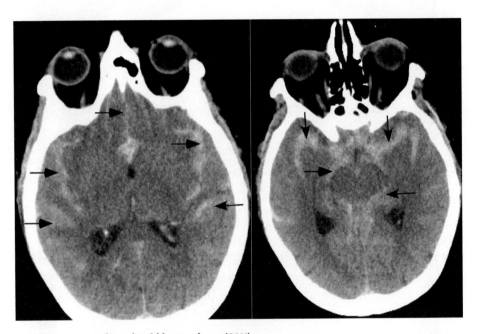

**FIGURE 1-7. Subarachnoid hemorrhage (SAH).**

Axial CT demonstrates high-density fluid layering along the bilateral cortical sulci, sylvian fissures, interhemispheric fissure, and basilar cisterns, all consistent with an SAH.

## Contusions (Fig. 1-8)

### LOCATION

Most common in the cortex of the frontal, temporal lobe and dorsal lateral midbrain.

### CAUSE

Direct impact of the brain with the overlying skull.

### CT FINDINGS

- Multiple hyperdense focal rounded lesions surrounded by low attenuation edema in characteristic locations
- Intraventricular hemorrhage is seen in 1% to 5% of patients with contusions.

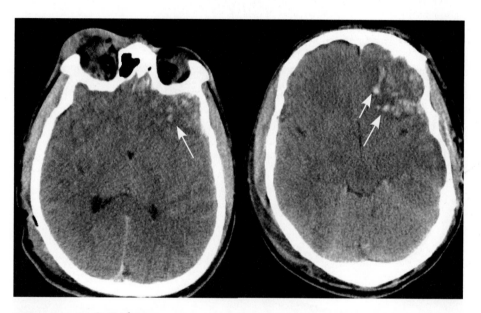

**FIGURE 1-8. Contusions.**

Focal punctate areas of high density (white arrows) in the bilateral inferior frontal lobes and left temporal lobe with surrounding low-attenuation changes. Findings are consistent with multiple contusions with surrounding edema.

### Diffuse Axonal Injury (DAI) (Fig. 1-9)

#### LOCATION

- Gray/white junctions
- Basal ganglia
- Corpus callosum
- Dorsal brain stem

DAI is the most common cause of posttraumatic vegetative state.

#### CAUSE

Acceleration/deceleration forces to the underlying brain, which cause injury to the axon. Typically seen after a high-speed motor vehicle accident.

#### CT FINDINGS

Multiple 4-mm to 5-mm hyperdense punctate lesions surrounded by edema (low attenuation) in the locations noted above. The extent of brain involvement is better seen on MRI since nonhemorrhagic lesions will also be seen, which may not be appreciated on CT.

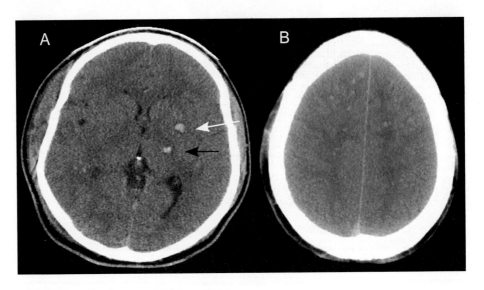

**FIGURE 1-9.  Diffuse axonal injury (DAI).**

High-attenuation changes in the left basal ganglia (white arrow), internal capsule (black arrow) (A), and gray/white junctions (B). Findings are all consistent with DAI.

## Types of Herniation

Key is knowing the cisterns.

### 1. SUBFALCINE HERNIATION (FIG. 1-10)

#### DEFINITION

Cingulate gyrus displaced under the falx cerebri.

#### CAUSE

Space-occupying lesion in the frontal or parietal lobe.

#### CT FINDINGS

- Draw a straight line from the septum pellucidum to the falx on an axial image and check if there is a midline shift.
- Shift of the third ventricle

This is the most common form of brain herniation.

Subfalcine herniation can be associated with an anterior cerebral artery (ACA) infarct.

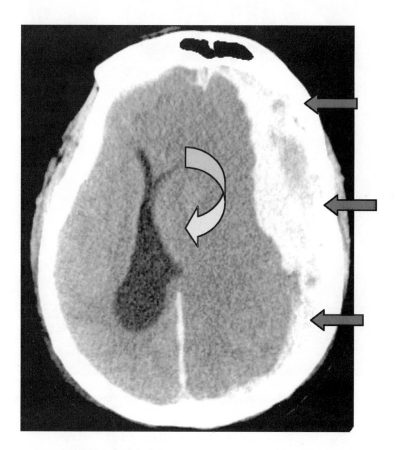

**FIGURE 1-10. Subfalcine herniation.**

Left hemispheric subdural hematoma (solid arrows) causing left-to-right midline shift with compression of the left lateral ventricle (curved arrow). Findings are consistent with a subfalcine herniation due to a subdural hematoma.

HIGH-YIELD FACTS

Neuroradiology

## 2. UNCAL HERNIATION (FIG. 1-11)

### DEFINITION

Displacement of the uncus medially

### CAUSE

Space-occupying mass in the brain results in herniation of the uncus medially.

### CT FINDINGS

- **Early:** Effacement of the ipsilateral suprasellar cistern
- **Late:** Complete effacement

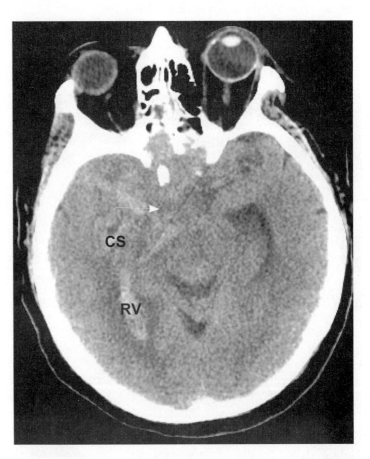

**FIGURE 1-11. Early uncal herniation on the right with effacement of the ipsilateral suprasellar cistern (arrow).**

There is acute hemorrhage in the right lateral ventricle (marked RV) and right cerebral sulci (marked CS).

### 3. Cerebellar Tonsillar Herniation (Fig. 1-12)

***Definition***

Downward herniation of the cerebellar tonsils

***Cause***

A space-occupying lesion in the posterior fossa, such as a tumor, or an Arnold-Chiari malformation

***CT Findings***

Effacement of the cisterna magna

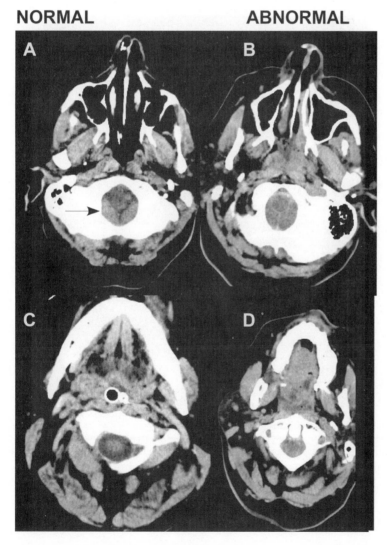

**NORMAL**          **ABNORMAL**

**FIGURE 1-12. Cerebellar tonsillar herniation.**

(A) Normal foramen magnum (arrow) and comparison with cerebellar herniation (B); (C) normal cervical spinal canal; (D) increased soft tissue around the chord. Findings are due to cerebellar herniation to the level of C1.

### Hydrocephalus

COMMUNICATING HYDROCEPHALUS (FIG. 1-13)

#### *DEFINITION*

Ventricles are markedly enlarged relative to the cortical sulci.

#### *CAUSE*

Decreased absorption of CSF

#### *CT FINDINGS*

Entire ventricular system is enlarged.

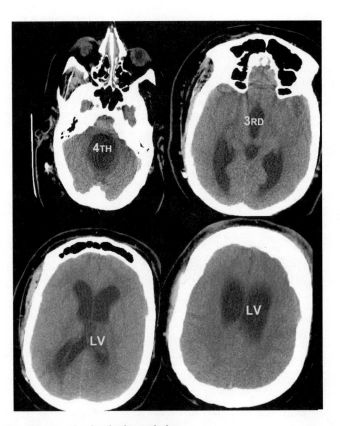

**FIGURE 1-13. Communicating hydrocephalus.**

Marked enlargement of the lateral left, third, and fourth ventricles consistent with communicating hydrocephalus.

## NONCOMMUNICATING HYDROCEPHALUS (FIG. 1-14)

### CAUSE

Blockage of cerebrospinal fluid (CSF) flow.

### CT FINDINGS

Only certain parts of the ventricular system are dilated; the rest is normal caliber.

The most common causes of hydrocephalus are meningitis and subarachnoid hemorrhage.

The most common cause of isolated hydrocephalus in children is congenital aqueductal stenosis.

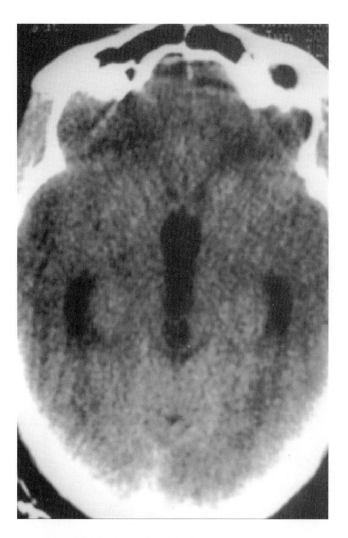

**FIGURE 1-14. Noncommunicating hydrocephalus.**

Enlargement of the lateral and third ventricle with effacement of the fourth ventricle consistent with noncommunicating hydrocephalus.

Increased risk of mass effect is seen between 3 and 5 days after infarction (ischemic stroke).

Hemorrhagic transformation may occur from 4 to 10 days after infarction (ischemic stroke).

## Stroke

### *CT FINDINGS*

- See Figure 1-15 for vascular supply of brain territories.
- Early CT findings: A CT can be normal within 24 hours. However, there are three early findings (< 24 hours) noted in an acute stroke that you should look for:
  - **Hyperdense middle cerebral artery (MCA) or ACA sign:** Due to a clot in the MCA or ACA, the MCA or ACA will appear hyperdense. This is a rare finding, but when it is present with associated symptoms, it is highly specific for an MCA or ACA stroke.
  - **Loss of gray/white differentiation.** Early on, this is first seen in the insular cortex.
  - **Mass effect:** Mild obliteration of sulci, adjacent ventricles, and subarachnoid space
- Late CT findings (24 hours to 21 days): Hypoattenuations seen in the MCA territory

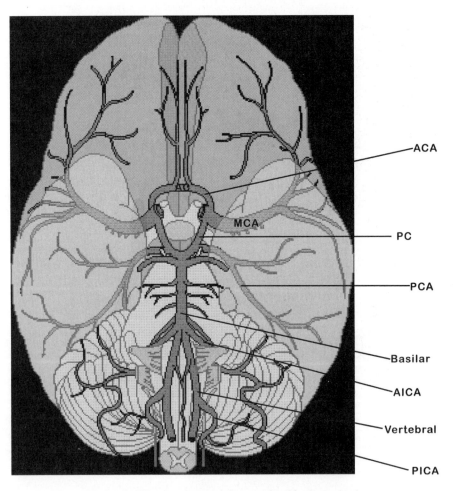

**FIGURE 1-15. Circle of Willis showing vascular supply of brain territories.**

## MCA Infarct (Fig. 1-16)

### *LOCATION*

In the MCA distribution including most of the basal ganglia, posterior lateral parietal, lateral occipital, and temporal lobe.

### *CAUSE*

Most commonly due to emboli secondary to arthrosclerosis in the internal carotid artery (ICA) and common carotid artery (CCA).

### *CT FINDINGS*

- **Early MCA stroke (0–24 hours):** Two specific signs:
  - **Hyperdense MCA sign:** Due to a clot in the MCA, the MCA will appear hyperdense.
  - **Loss of insular stripe:** Loss of gray/white differentiation in the insular cortex

Mass effect progresses the most during the first 3 days after an MCA infarct.

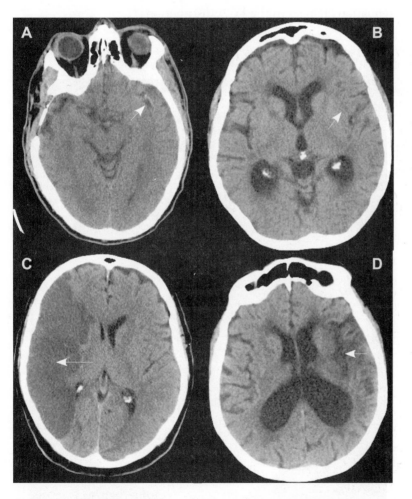

**FIGURE 1-16. MCA infarct.**

(A) Hyperdense MCA sign with increased attenuation in the left MCA distribution; (B) loss of the insular stripe on the left compared to normal on the right; (C) wedge shaped, well-defined, low-attenuation changes consistent with a subacute infarct; (D) very low density on the left with preservation of the sulci, and associated encephalomalacia of the adjacent lateral ventricle, consistent with a chronic infarct.

- **Subacute MCA stroke (2–21 days):** Focal wedge-shaped area of low attenuation in the MCA distribution
- **Chronic MCA stroke (> 21 days):** Progressive increase in hypoattenuation associated with ex vacuo dilatation of the adjacent subarachnoid spaces and ventricles called encephalomalacia.

### PCA Infarct (Fig. 1-17)

#### LOCATION

In the PCA distribution including the midbrain, medial temporal, and occipital lobes.

#### CAUSES

- Usually from an embolic source
- May also be seen due to uncal herniation

#### CT FINDINGS

Low-attenuation changes in the PCA distribution

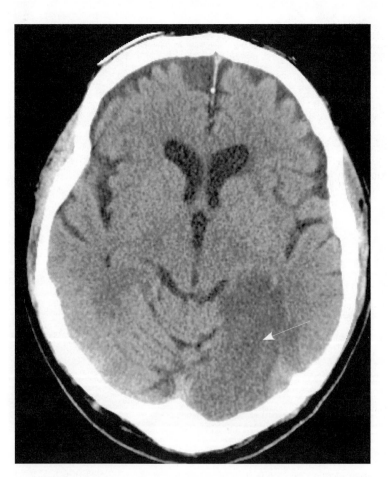

**FIGURE 1-17. Low-attenuation changes in the left PCA distribution, consistent with a PCA infarct (arrow).**

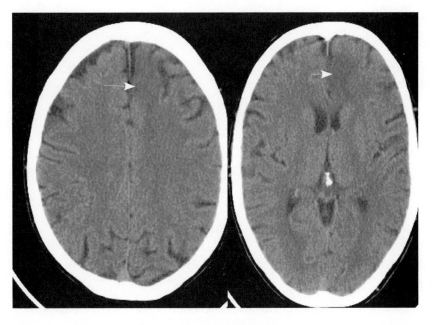

FIGURE 1-18. Low-attenuation changes in the left ACA distribution consistent with an ACA infarct (arrow).

## ACA Infarct (Fig. 1-18)

### LOCATION

ACA distribution including the medial aspects of the frontal and parietal lobe, corpus callosum, and rostral portions of the basal ganglia.

### CAUSES

- Usually 2° to 1° vessel disease and not emboli
- May also be due to subfalcine herniation (see Fig. 1-18)

### CT FINDINGS

Hypoattenuation in the ACA distribution

ACA infarct is the least common type of infarct.

ACA infarct is associated with ICA occlusion.

## Watershed Infarct

### LOCATION

Occurs between the ACA and MCA, and MCA and PCA

### CAUSES

- Decreased perfusion between the major vascular territories, which receives blood from the distal branches of the two neighboring arteries
- If bilateral: Hypoxia, hypotension, cardiac arrest
- If unilateral: Possible occlusion or stenosis of ipsilateral ICA

### CT FINDINGS

Low-attenuation changes in a wedge-shaped pattern extending from the corners of lateral ventricles

### Intracerebral Hemorrhage (ICH) (Fig. 1-19)

#### *LOCATION*

Commonly involves putamen, external capsule, thalamus, pons, cerebellum, and subcortical white matter

#### *CAUSES*

- Acute hypertension
- Trauma
- Ruptured aneurysm
- Vascular malformations
- Amyloid
- Anticoagulation
- Neoplasia
- Cocaine

#### *CT FINDINGS*

Focal area of high density of the above described characteristic locations

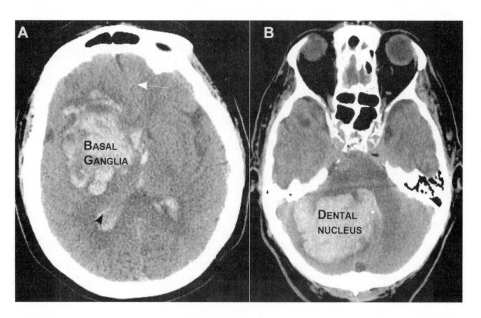

**FIGURE 1-19.** Intracerebral hemorrhage.

(A) Axial CT shows an acute hemorrhage involving the right basal ganglia with extension into the intraventricular system (black arrow) and right to left midline shift (white arrow). (B) 7-cm intraparenchymal hemorrhage centered within the right dentate nucleus.

- The most important diagnostic measure is to determine if the mass is extra-axial or intra-axial (Fig. 1-20).
  - An **extra-axial mass** arises from outside the brain. This includes the arachnoid, meninges, dural sinuses, skull, etc.
  - An **intra-axial mass** arises from within the brain.
- The key to differentiate between the two is "white matter buckling." This is created by an extra-axial mass pushing the white matter inward and the gray/white interface is still defined. On the other hand, an intra-axial mass expands the white matter and effaces the gray/white interface.

Extra-axial            Intra-axial

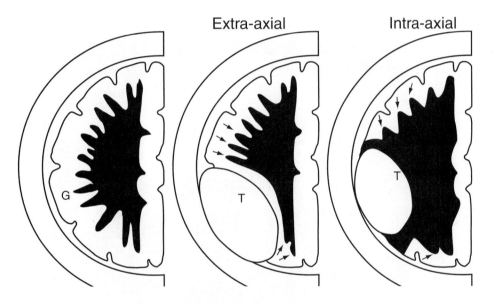

**FIGURE 1-20.** **Location of intracranial tumor: intra-axial vs. extra-axial.**

GBM is the most common intra-axial tumor and the most malignant type of glial tumor.

GBM is the most common 1° hemorrhagic tumor; oligodendroglioma is second most common.

**Intra-axial Tumors**

## GLIOBLASTOMA MULTIFORME (GBM) (FIG. 1-21)

### *LOCATION*

Most common location is in the deep white matter of the frontal lobe.

### *NONCONTRAST CT FINDINGS*

- Heterogenous, lobulated with surrounding edema
- Hemorrhage and necrosis are also common findings.

### *CONTRAST-ENHANCED CT FINDINGS*

Irregular, nodular, ringlike enhancement

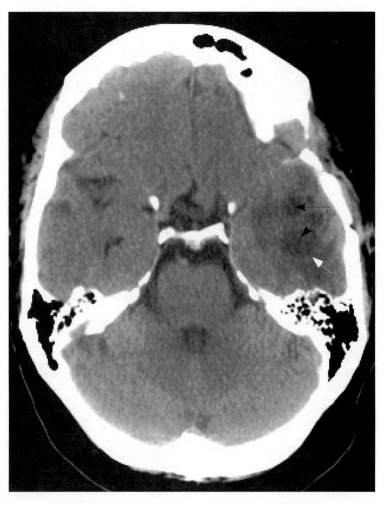

**FIGURE 1-21. Heterogenous, low-attenuation lobulated mass (black arrows) in the left middle cranial fossa with surrounding edema (white arrow) in a patient with biopsy proven GBM.**

## HEMANGIOBLASTOMA (FIG. 1-22)

### LOCATION

Most common in the cerebellar hemispheres

### CT FINDINGS

Well-defined cystic mass with an enhancing mural nodule

Hemangioblastoma is the most common 1° intra-axial neoplasm of the posterior fossa in adults and 4% to 20% occur in association with von Hippel–Lindau disease.

Toxoplasmosis is the most common brain tumor in AIDS patients.

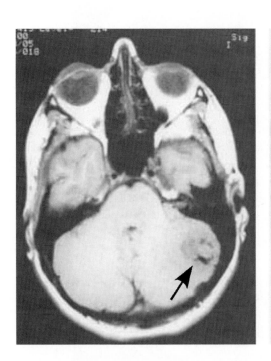
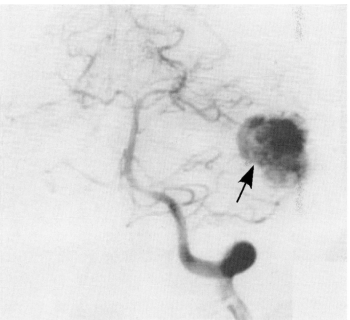

**FIGURE 1-22.** Left panel depicts MRI of hemangioblastoma in the left posterior fossa (arrow). Right panel depicts an angiogram of the same hypervascular hemangioblastoma.

(Reproduced, with permission, from accessmedicine.com, McGraw-Hill, 2008.)

Ring-enhancing lesion differential:
- Tumor
- Abscess
- Resolving hematoma

Whenever you see a lesion spreading across the corpus callosum, it is one of four diseases:
- Lymphoma
- GBM
- Demyelinating disease
- Trauma

## PRIMARY LYMPHOMA (FIG. 1-23)

### LOCATION

Deep gray or white matter; can characteristically cross the corpus callosum.

### CT FINDINGS

- Immunocompetent patients: Slightly high attenuation mass with negligible mass effect. It enhances avidly with IV contrast.
- Immunosuppressed patients: Multiple ring-enhancing lesions; main differential is toxoplasmosis.

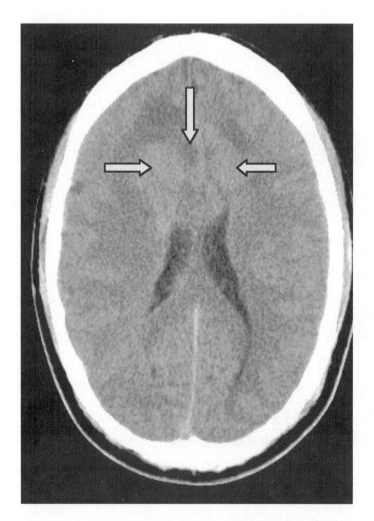

**FIGURE 1-23. Slightly high attenuation lobulated mass that crosses both cerebral hemispheres above the lateral ventricles in a patient with biopsy-proven lymphoma (arrows).**

## Metastasis (Fig. 1-24)

### Location

Gray/white junctions; majority are supratentorial.

### CT Findings

- Isodense, hypodense, or hyperdense (if hemorrhagic) mass at gray/white junction
- Surrounding low-attenuation edema
- Nodular, ring, or focal enhancement

> Brain metastases most commonly come from lung, breast, or skin (melanoma).

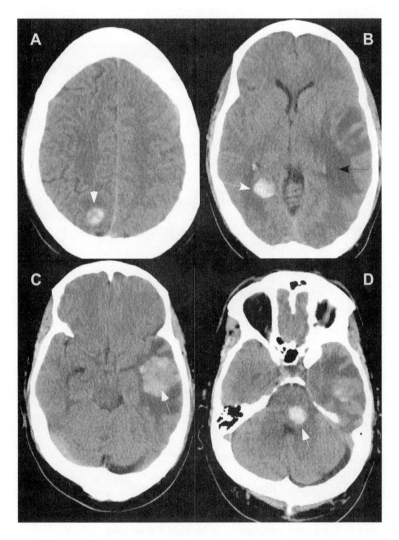

**FIGURE 1-24.** Noncontrast CT demonstrating multiple hemorrhagic intracranial metastases.

Metastatic melanoma in the (A) right parietal lobe, (B) right occipital, (C) left temporal lobe, and (D) brain stem. In addition, the black arrow in plate (B) shows a surrounding peritumoral edema.

### Extra-axial Tumors (Fig. 1-25)

#### MENINGIOMA

##### *LOCATION*

- In the parasagittal or convexity location 50% of the time
- Other locations: Sphenoid wing (20%), olfactory groove (10%), parasellar (10%), also the spine.

#### *CT FINDINGS*

Hyperdense masses with extreme homogenous enhancement. Key to diagnosis is the broad dural base.

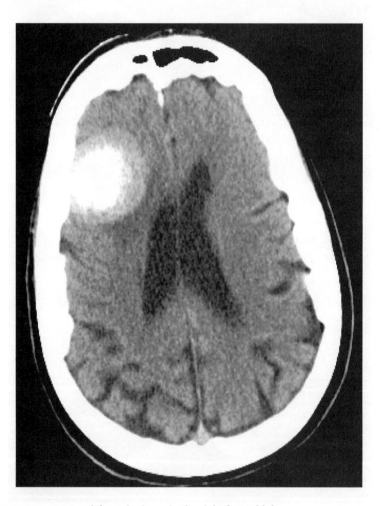

**FIGURE 1-25. Extra-axial meningioma in the right frontal lobe.**

## Arachnoid Cyst (Fig. 1-26)

### Location

Sylvian fissure (50%), suprasellar (10%), quadrigeminal plate cistern (10%), cerebellar pontine angle (5% to 10%)

### Imaging Findings

- Well-defined, low-attenuation CSF density mass.
- Signal parallels CSF on all sequences in MRI.
- May produce scalloping of the adjacent bone.

- The main differential for an arachnoid cyst is an epidermoid cyst.
- An arachnoid cyst on MRI demonstrates no restriction (appearing dark) on diffusion-weighted imaging, whereas an epidermoid cyst does have restricted diffusion (appearing bright).

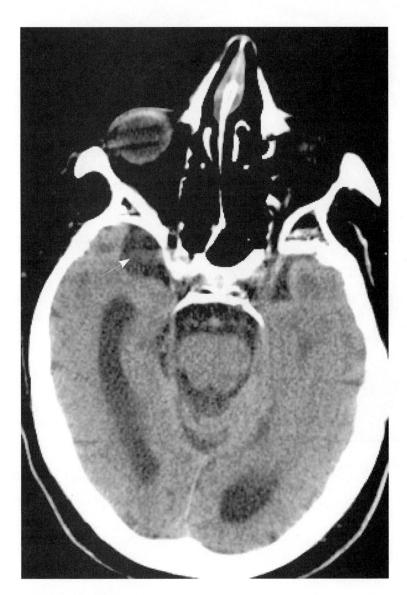

**FIGURE 1-26. Arachnoid cyst (arrow).**

A colloid cyst can cause acute hydrocephalus, which can result in sudden death.

## COLLOID CYST (FIG. 1-27)

### *LOCATION*

Anterior third ventricle

### *CT FINDINGS*

Usually high-attenuation spherical mass in the anterior third ventricle; may result in obstructive hydrocephalus

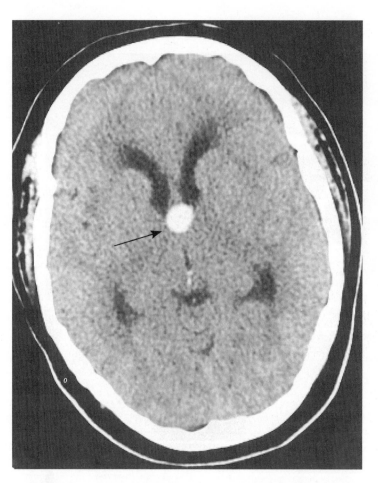

**FIGURE 1-27. Colloid cyst (arrow).**

## Cerebral Abscess (Fig. 1-28)

### LOCATION

Most common in the temporal, frontal, parietal lobes

### CAUSE

May develop after trauma, surgery, sinus or dental infection

### IMAGING FINDINGS

- Variable
- CT: Usually, a thin-walled ring enhancing mass surrounding low attenuation edematous changes
- MRI: Bright on diffusion-weighted imaging (DWI), and dark on apparent diffusion coefficient (ADC).

When cerebral abscess is secondary to hematogenous spread, the MCA territory is commonly involved.

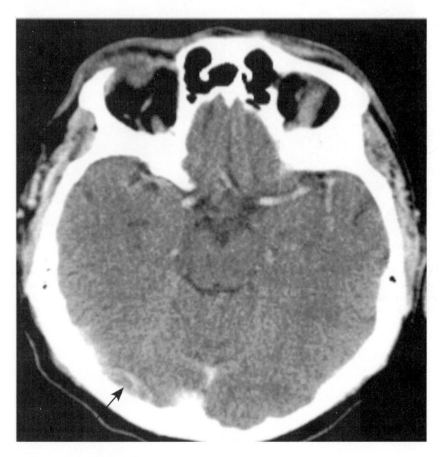

**FIGURE 1-28. Cerebral abscess (arrow).**

HIGH-YIELD FACTS

Neuroradiology

### Herpes Encephalitis (Fig. 1-29)

#### LOCATION

Most common in temporal lobes

#### CAUSES

- Adults: Secondary to reactivation of latent herpes simplex type 1
- Neonates: Secondary to herpes simplex type 2. The neonate acquires this after exposure through the birth canal when the mother has an active infection.

#### CT FINDINGS

- CT is usually normal in acute stage.
- Usually areas of decreased attenuation in one or both temporal lobes
- Hemorrhagic transformation can occur.

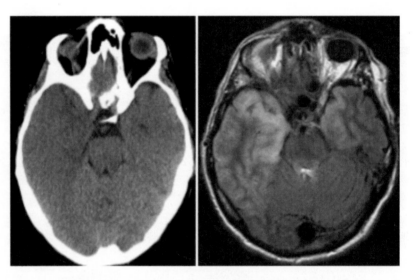

FIGURE 1-29. Noncontrast CT demonstrates low attenuation in the right middle cranial fossa. MRI of the same patients demonstrates increased T2 signal in both temporal lobes consistent with Herpes Encephalitis.

HIGH-YIELD FACTS

Neuroradiology

## Meningitis

### LOCATION

Nonspecific

### CAUSES

Most common bacterial causes:

- Adults: *Streptococcus pneumoniae*
- Children: *Haemophilus influenzae*
- Young adults: *Neisseria meningitidis*

### IMAGING FINDINGS

- Nonspecific
- Diffuse cerebral edema
- MRI has a greater sensitivity than CT and may show dural, leptomeningeal, or ependymal enhancement.

## Sinusitis (Fig. 1-30)

### LOCATION

Frontal, maxillary, sphenoid, and ethmoid sinus

### CAUSE

Most commonly due to viral upper respiratory tract infections

### CT FINDINGS

- Opacification of the sinus(es)
- Air-fluid levels
- Mucosal thickening

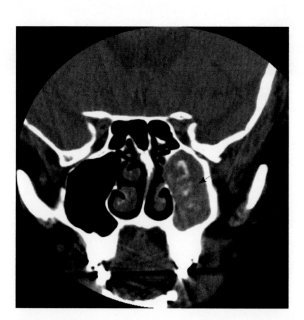

**FIGURE 1-30. CT of the paranasal sinues shows left maxillary sinusitis with calcified material (arrow) within suggestive of chronicall inspissated mucus.**

A calcified choroid plexus or calcified pineal gland is a normal finding—do not mistake for blood! Could check on bone window to make sure it is calcification.

### Calcified Choroid Plexus (Fig. 1-31)

#### *LOCATION*

Within the choroid plexus

#### *CT FINDINGS*

High-density calcification within the choroid plexus

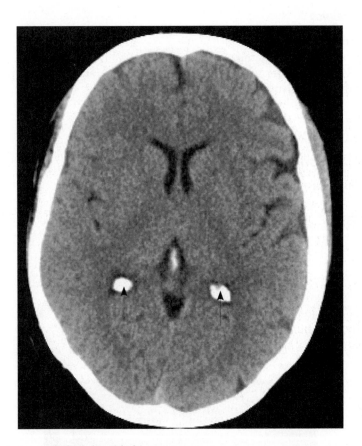

FIGURE 1-31. **Calcified choroid plexus.**

## Calcified Pineal Gland (Fig. 1-32)

### LOCATION

Pineal gland

### CT FINDINGS

Focal high density within the pineal gland

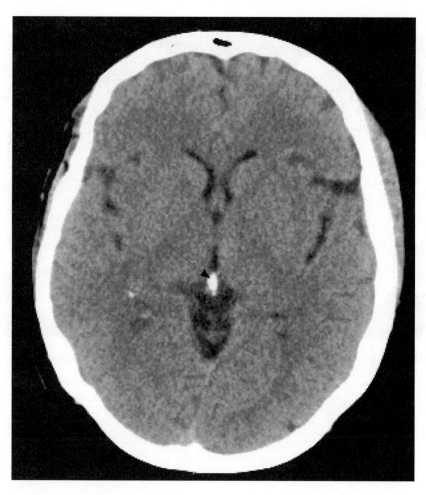

FIGURE 1-32. Calcified pineal gland.

Small vessel ischemic change is a normal age-related finding.

## Small Vessel Ischemic Change (Fig. 1-33)

### *LOCATION*

Periventricular.

### *CT FINDINGS*

- Low-attenuation perventricular changes.
- Look also for prominent lateral ventricles, cortical sulci.

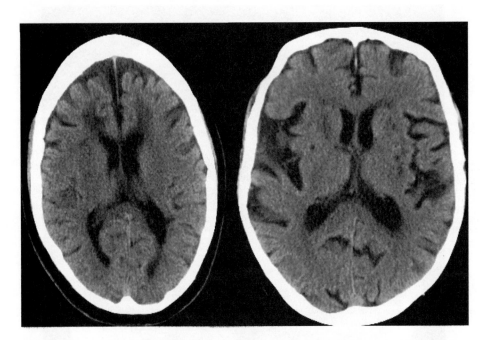

**FIGURE 1-33. Age-related periventricular ischemic changes, with age-related cerebral atrophy.**

## Multiple Sclerosis (Fig. 1-34)

### *Location*

Most common in periventricular white matter, corpus callosum.

### *Imaging Findings*

- T2WI/fluid attenuation inversion recovery (FLAIR) MRI: Bilateral ovoid hyperintense lesions; incomplete peripheral enhancement
- CT: May see patchy periventricular areas of low attenuation

Multiple sclerosis:
- Most common demyelinating disorder
- More common in women
- MRI is the most sensitive test, particularly the FLAIR sequence.

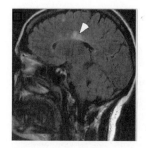

**FIGURE 1-34. MRI in a patient with multiple sclerosis.**

Note: High-signal intensity in FLAIR images in periventricular white matter, this represents "Dawson's Finger."

# Chest Radiology

- **Advantages**: Quick test that can usually identify pathological processes such as pneumonia, congestive heart failure, etc.
- **Disadvantages**: Not as comprehensive as a chest CT. For example, it cannot rule out processes such as a pulmonary embolus.
- **When to order**: Common indications include shortness of breath, chest pain.

### How to Read a Chest X-ray

You must first check for four things:

- **Penetration:** Good penetration is when the intervertebral disk spaces and the vasculature can be visualized.
- **Rotation:** Draw a vertical line through the spinous processes of the thoracic vertebrae and a horizontal line through the medial margins of the clavicular heads to assess rotation. Where these lines intersect, equal distance should be noted on each side between the spinous process and the medial clavicular head on each side of the spinous processes.
- **Inspiration**: Good inspiration is counting 10–11 posterior ribs.
- **Motion:** Outline of the chest structures should be sharp. This is assessed by noting well-defined borders of the chest structures such as the heart and diaphragm.

Systematic approach to chest x-ray interpretation* (Fig. 2-1):

- **A**irway: Check to see if the trachea is midline.
- **B**one: Look for fractures.
- **C**ardiac: Look to see if the heart is enlarged.
- **D**iaphragm: Check for free air under the diaphragm and pleural effusions.
- **E**xtras: Identify all tubes and lines.
- **F**ields of the lung: Check the lung parenchyma for an atelectasis or consolidation.

**CHEST X-RAY**

- The first thing you should check on a chest x-ray is the patient's name.
- On an AP view you cannot diagnose cardiomegaly since anterior structures are magnified. There is an apparent increase in vascularity and heart size in a supine anteroposterior chest radiograph. See Figure 2-2.
- Overexposure causes a film to be black.
- The four basic radiographic densities: bone, water, fat, and air. The denser the body part, the whiter it will appear on film. For example, since bone is most dense, it will appear the whitest on an x-ray. Air is the least dense, and thus will appear black on an x-ray.

**HIGH-YIELD FACTS**

**Chest Radiology**

---

*Adapted from Ayala C, Spellberg B: *Boards and Wards*. Philadelphia: Lippincott Williams & Wilkins, 2006.

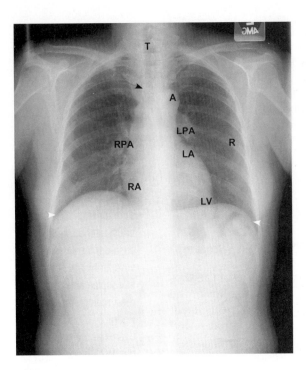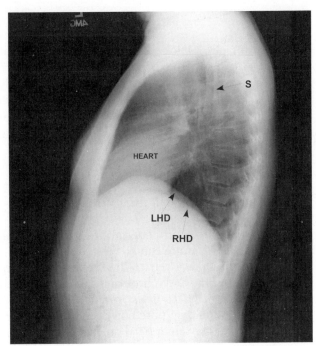

**FIGURE 2-1. A normal PA and lateral chest X-ray.**

T: trachea; A: aortic knob; RPA: right pulmonary artery; LPA, left pulmonary artery; R, rib; LA, left atrium; RA, right atrium; LV, left ventricle; LHD, left hemidiaphragm; RHD, right hemidiaphragm; S, scapula. On PA view, note superior vena cava (black arrow) and costophrenic angles (white arrows).

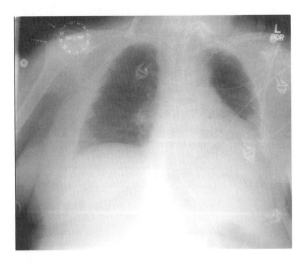

**FIGURE 2-2. AP and supine chest radiograph depicting apparent increase in vascularity and heart size.**

CT density is expressed in Hounsfield Units (HUs). The scanner is calibrated so that water is zero HU. Typical values are: bone = 350, muscle = 40, water = 0, fat = –120, lung = –800 (Fig. 2-3).

- **Advantages:** The main advantage over plain x-rays is its ability to produce cross-sectional images without the limitations of overlapping of structures that occurs on the chest x-ray, and the greater contrast sensitivity of CT images that can show the normal and abnormal pathologic processes within the chest.
- **Disadvantages:** Increased radiation dose, and if contrast is given, there is a risk of renal problems and anaphylactic reaction in some patients.

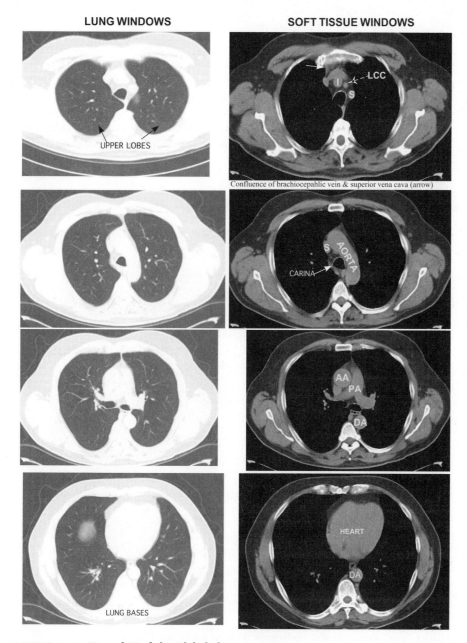

**FIGURE 2-3. Normal CT of chest labeled.**

AA, ascending aorta; DA, descending aorta; PA, pulmonary artery; LCC, left common carotid; S. superior venacava.

51

- **Silhouette sign:** An interface is not visible when two areas of similar density overlap (see Figure 2-8).

- **Golden S sign:** When the horizontal fissure in the right upper lobe takes on an "S" shaped appearance, this is indicative that an underlying mass is present (see Figure 2-4).

- **Luftsichel sign:** The lucency you see around the aortic arch due to LLL hyperinflation. This represents significant volume loss in the left upper lobe (LUL).

- **When to order:** Numerous indications, which include to further evaluate a pulmonary nodule seen on a chest x-ray or to rule out a pulmonary embolus.

## ▶ ATELECTASIS

### Complete Atelectasis (Collapse)

#### *CAUSES*

Volume loss within the lung due to numerous causes such as a mucous plug, aspirated foreign body, carcinoma, pneumothorax, radiation, benign tumor, etc.

#### *CHEST X-RAY FINDINGS*

- Upper lobes collapse in an upward, medial, and anterior direction.
- Indirect signs of collapse include a displaced fissure, shift of structures to ipsilateral side, and loss of definition of adjacent soft tissues of similar density (silhouette sign) (Fig. 2-8).
- When the right middle lobe (RML) collapses it obscures the right heart border on a PA or AP view. Middle lobe collapse is best appreciated on the lateral view.

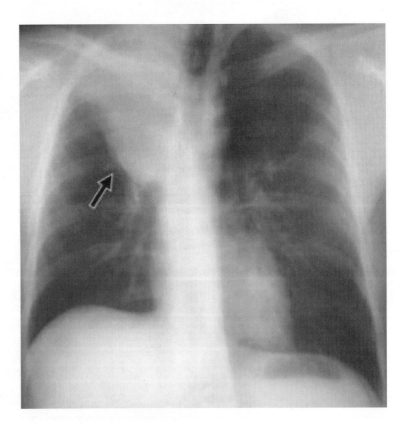

**FIGURE 2-4. Complete RUL atelectasis "Golden S sign" on PA CXR.**

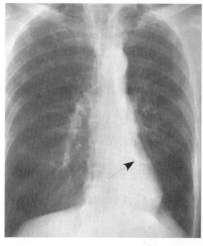
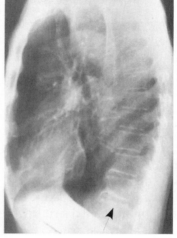
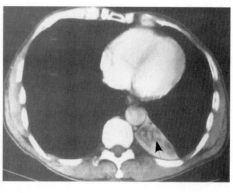

**FIGURE 2-5. LLL collapse on PA and lateral CXR and CT.**

(Reproduced, with permission from: Chen MY, Pope TL, Ott DJ: *Basic Radiology*. New York: McGraw-Hill, 2008: 80.)

- When the lingula collapses it obscures the left heart border on a PA or AP view. On a lateral view there will be a focal white triangle formed by the minor and major fissure.
- Both right lower lobe (RLL) and left lower lobe (LLL) collapse posteriorly, medially, and downward. The diaphragm border will be obliterated on the frontal view (Fig. 2-5).

## Linear Atelectasis (Fig. 2-6)

### CAUSES

- Typically seen after recent surgery
- Rib fractures in a patient who has difficulty breathing

### CHEST X-RAY FINDINGS

Horizontal focal area of increased density usually in the middle or lower lungs

- Central obstruction in children is usually due to a mucous plug or aspirated foreign body.
- Central obstruction in an adult over the age of 40 is most likely due to bronchogenic carcinoma.

Linear atelectasis is also known as platelike or discoid atelectasis.

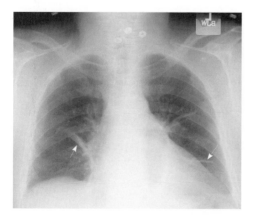

**FIGURE 2-6. CXR demonstrating linear atelectasis (arrows) in right middle zone and left lower zone.**

### CAUSES

- Bacteria
- Viruses
- Fungi

### CHEST X-RAY FINDINGS

- Figure 2-7 depicts a right upper lobe (RUL) pneumonia
- Area of increased opacity, sometimes described as "fluffy" (Fig. 2-11)
- Fissures do not move
- No shift in mediastinal structures
- May see air bronchogram sign (Fig. 2-8)

### CT FINDINGS

- Figure 2-10 depicts a LLL pneumonia

Other causes of alveolar infiltrate (besides pneumonia):
- Blood (hemorrhage)
- Fluid (fluid)
- Cells (tumor)

HIGH-YIELD FACTS

Chest Radiology

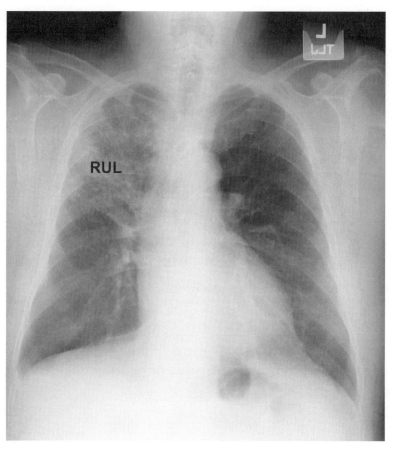

FIGURE 2-7. CXR demonstrating RUL pneumonia.

**Air bronchogram sign:**
When air is seen in the intrapulmonary bronchi due to surrounding consolidation by a pathological process outlying the bronchus. This may be seen in pneumonia, pulmonary edema, pulmonary infarcts, and certain lung diseases (Fig. 2-8).

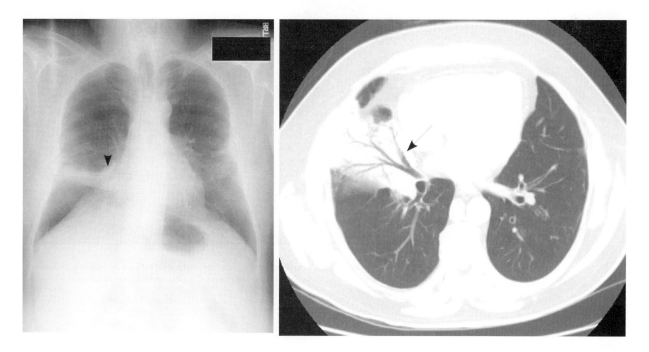

FIGURE 2-8. CXR demonstrating RML pneumonia.

Note increased opacity in RML abutting the right heart border on CXR (silhouette sign). Note air bronchogram on CT (arrow).

**Spine sign:** On lateral view, thoracic vertebral bodies should get darker as you move down toward the abdomen. If they get whiter, be suspicious of a lower lobe infiltrate (Fig. 2-9).

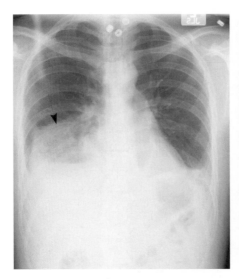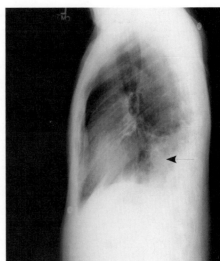

**FIGURE 2-9. CXR demonstrating RLL pneumonia.**

Note spine sign on the lateral view.

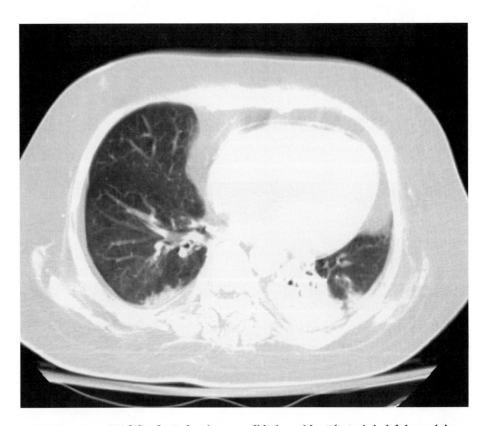

**FIGURE 2-10. CT of the chest showing consolidation with atelectasis in left lower lobe.**

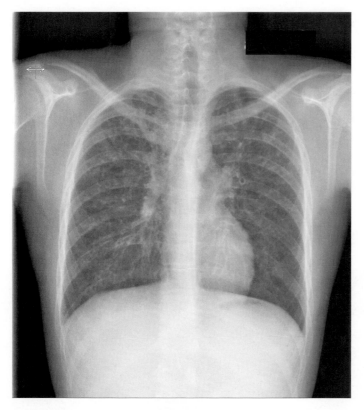

**FIGURE 2-11.  Bilateral nodular interstitial infiltrates.**

Findings likely due to atypical mycobacterial infection.

If you are not sure if a nodule is benign, the first thing you should do is to compare to old films/CT. If the nodule has been present more than 2 years with no change in size, it is likely benign. Another option is to obtain a CT scan for further evaluation.

### Benign Pulmonary Nodules

#### CAUSES

- Most likely due to a granuloma (Fig. 2-12).
- Other causes include hamartoma (Fig. 2-13), AV malformation, and septic embolus.

#### CHEST X-RAY FINDINGS

Round, well-defined with smooth borders, and central calcification.

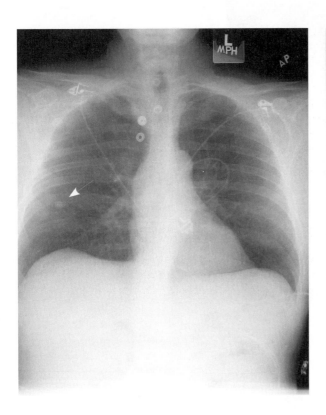
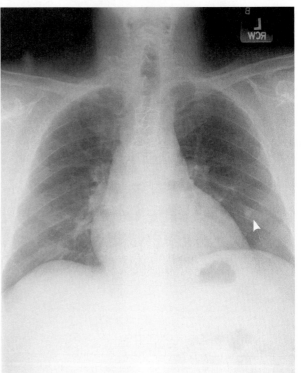

**FIGURE 2-12. CXRs demonstrating calcified granulomas.**

HIGH-YIELD FACTS

Chest Radiology

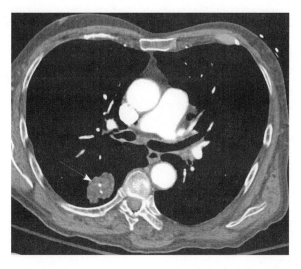

**FIGURE 2-13.** CT depicting popcorn calcification in the RLL typical of hamartoma or benign lesion.

## Malignant Pulmonary Nodule

### *CAUSE*

Metastatic lesions or a primary neoplasm (Fig. 2-14).

### *CHEST X-RAY FINDINGS*

- Usually greater than 3 cm in diameter
- Irregular shape and borders
- If spiculated, there is a 90% chance of malignancy
- No central calcification

- A CT scan should be suggested for further evaluation if a suspicious nodule is seen on x-ray.
- Most common places to miss tumors are the apices of the lung and behind the heart.

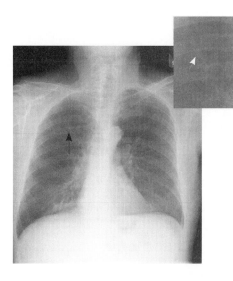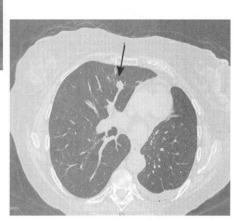

**FIGURE 2-14.** Left panel is a CXR depicting an indeterminate nodule in the RUL. Right panel is a CT demonstrating a spiculated nodule in the right mid lung consistent with biopsy proven carcinoma.

### Malignant Cavity (Fig. 2-15)

***CAUSE***

Squamous cell tumors that tend to cavitate

***CHEST X-RAY FINDINGS***

- Thick walled, greater than 4 mm
- Irregular, thick inner wall
- May have an air-fluid level

Use the contour of the inner wall to help differentiate an abscess from a malignancy. Wall is usually smooth in an abscess, and irregular in malignancy.

### Abscess Cavity (Fig. 2-16)

***CAUSE***

Toxins or necrotic pneumonias

***CHEST X-RAY FINDINGS***

- Thick walled, greater than 4 mm
- Smooth inner wall
- May have an air-fluid level

### Granuloma Cavity (Fig. 2-17)

***CAUSE***

Likely due to fungal infection, such as histoplasmosis, aspergillosis (Fig. 2-18) or lung hydatid disease (Fig. 2-19).

***CHEST X-RAY FINDINGS***

Thick or thin walled (less than 4 mm), but lack an air-fluid level.

Granuloma cavity: Most commonly a thin-walled cavity less than 4 mm with no air-fluid level.

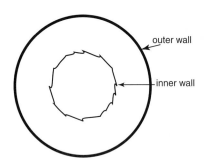

**FIGURE 2-15. Malignant cavity.**

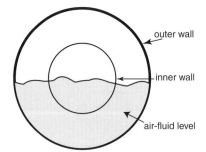

**FIGURE 2-16. Abscess cavity.**

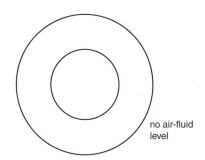

**FIGURE 2-17. Granuloma cavity.**

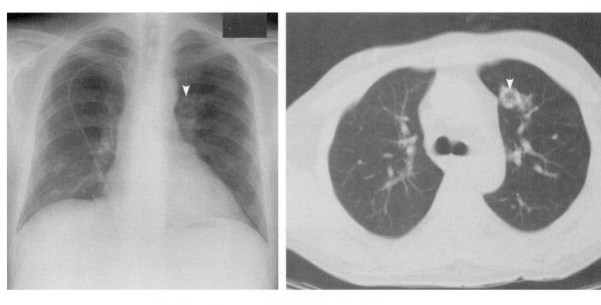

FIGURE 2-18. CXR in a posttransplant leukemic patient with aspergillosis showing patchy infiltrates in the right base with cavitary lesion in the left midzone (arrow). Central line is noted in the SVC.

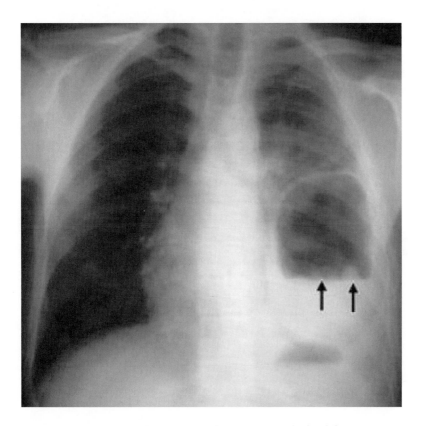

FIGURE 2-19. CXR showing classical water lily sign in lung hydatid disease.

Check to see if the bullous changes were present on previous x-ray. Since it is a chronic process, it would likely be seen on an old x-ray as opposed to a pneumothorax, which is an acute finding.

## Pulmonary Bullae

### CAUSE

Usually seen in emphysematous lungs (Fig. 2-20). They are thin-walled cystic spaces larger than 1 cm in diameter and found within the lung parenchyma.

### CHEST X-RAY FINDINGS

- A lucent, well-defined lesion within the lung
- Look for vessels that can sometimes be seen within the bullae.

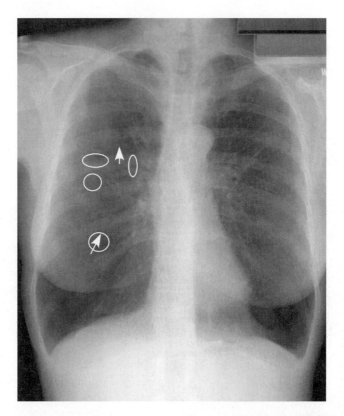

FIGURE 2-20. CXR depicting emphysematous changes in both lungs with bullous changes in the apices.

- There are a large number of diseases located in the mediastinum.
- They are classified based on their location in the anterior, middle, or posterior mediastinum.
- It is important to use the silhouette sign (when an air–soft tissue interface is lost due to a secondary process) to help determine its location.

## Anterior Mediastinal Mass (Fig. 2-21)

### CAUSES

4-T's:

- **T**hymoma
- **T**eratoma (germ cell tumors)
- **T**errible lymphoma
- **T**hyroid lesions

### CHEST X-RAY FINDINGS

- On a lateral view there will be increased opacity in the retrosternal space.
- On PA or AP view there will be increased opacity silhouetting the heart.

The most common anterior mediastinal mass is thymoma.

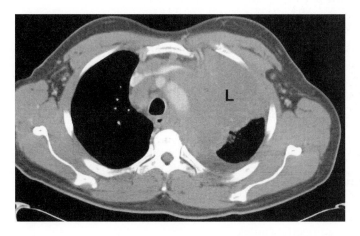
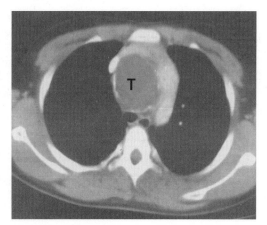

**FIGURE 2-21. Chest CT showing anterior mediastinal mass due to lymphoma (L, left panel), and Teratoma (T, right panel).**

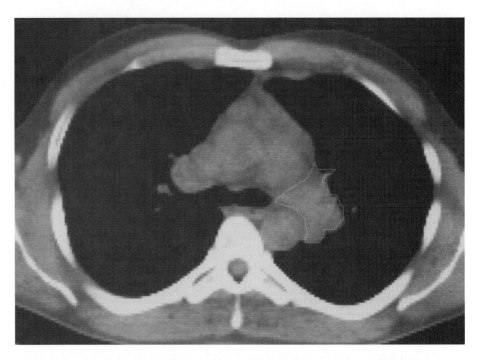

**FIGURE 2-22.** Chest CT shows a low-density, nonenhancing middle mediastinal mass (outline) posterior to great vessels and anterior to trachea.

Most common cause of a middle mediastinal mass is adenopathy.

## Middle Mediastinal Mass (Fig. 2-22)

### CAUSE

Adenopathy, duplication cyst, aortic aneurysm, hematoma, neoplasm, and esophageal lesions.

### CHEST X-RAY FINDINGS

Increased opacity silhouetting structures such as the aorta and pulmonary arteries in the middle mediastinum.

## Posterior Mediastinal Mass (Fig. 2-23)

### CAUSES

Usually secondary to neurogenic causes

- Neuroblastoma
- Neurofibroma
- Schwannomas
- Ganglioneuromas

Posterior mediastinal mass:
- If the patient is less than 2 years old, most likely malignant neuroblastoma.
- If between 18 and 20 years old, usually benign.

### IMAGING FINDINGS

- Increased opacity in the posterior mediastinum
- May cause an increase in size of the neural foramina (in case of neurogenic tumors)
- May see widened intercostal space posteriorly

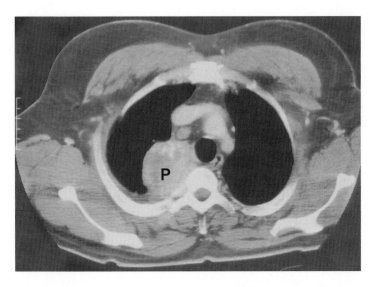

**FIGURE 2-23. Chest CT showing posterior mediastinal mass due to paraganglioma.**

## Cardiomegaly

### CAUSES

Numerous causes such as hypertension, renal failure, valvular lesions, cardiomyopathy, severe anemia, thyroid disorders, hemochromatosis, and amyloidosis.

### CHEST X-RAY FINDINGS

Measure from the most lateral borders of the heart and compare this width to the inner border of the widest part of the inner rib; if this ratio exceeds 50%, the diagnosis can be made.

## Congestive Heart Failure (CHF)

### STAGE I CHF (PROGRESSIVE CEPHALIZATION) (FIG. 2-24)

### CAUSE

Increased mean capillary wedge pressure 10–20 mm Hg

### CHEST X-RAY FINDINGS

Progressive cephalization, which means increased blood flow toward the top of the lung

Make sure that you are looking at a PA chest X-ray when diagnosing, cardiomegaly since the heart is magnified on an AP view.

Cephalization: Can only use this sign on an upright chest x-ray, not supine, since blood flow will redistribute.

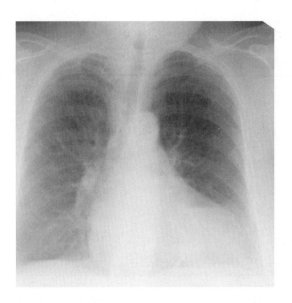

**FIGURE 2-24. CXR showing cardiomegaly with cephalization in a patient with pulmonary venous hypertension.**

Kerley B lines: Horizontal white lines at the lung bases extending from the periphery of the lung.

### STAGE 2 CHF (INTERSTITIAL EDEMA)

#### CAUSE

Increased mean capillary wedge pressure 20–25 mm Hg

#### CHEST X-RAY FINDINGS

Thin white lines due to interstitial edema, known as Kerley B lines

### STAGE 3 CHF (ALVEOLAR EDEMA)

#### CAUSE

Wedge pressure greater than 25 mm Hg

#### CHEST X-RAY FINDINGS

Increased opacity around the hila in a butterfly pattern referred to as "bat wings" appearance

## Stage 4 CHF (Chronic Pulmonary Venous Hypertension) (Fig. 2-25)

### Cause

Increased wedge pressure greater than 30 mm Hg

### Chest X-ray Findings

Bilateral interstitial infiltrates and bilateral pleural effusions.

If the patient doesn't have cardiomegaly, consider noncardiogenic causes of CHF such as head injury or drug overdose.

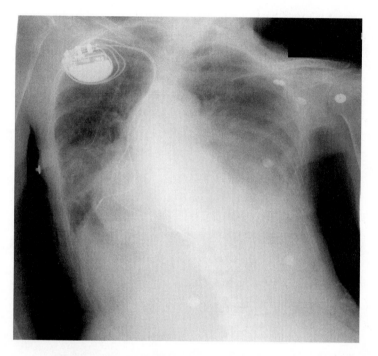

**FIGURE 2-25.** **CXR depicting cardiomegaly with bilateral interstitial infiltrates and bilateral pleural effusions, consistent with advanced CHF.**

Note also grossly scoliotic spine.

### Pleural Effusion (Fig. 2-26)

#### CAUSE

Pleural effusion can be caused by CHF, cirrhosis, nephrotic syndrome, trauma, cancer, pneumonia, tuberculosis, pulmonary embolism, tumor, trauma, collagen vascular disease, or atelectasis.

#### CHEST X-RAY FINDINGS

- PA chest x-ray: The lateral costophrenic angle will be blunted.
- Lateral view x-ray: The posterior costophrenic angle will be blunted.
- Lateral decubitus view: With patient on his/her side, a layer of fluid will be visible.

- At least 100 cc of pleural fluid should be present to be seen on an upright chest x-ray.
- As little as 5 cc of fluid can be detected on a decubitus view.

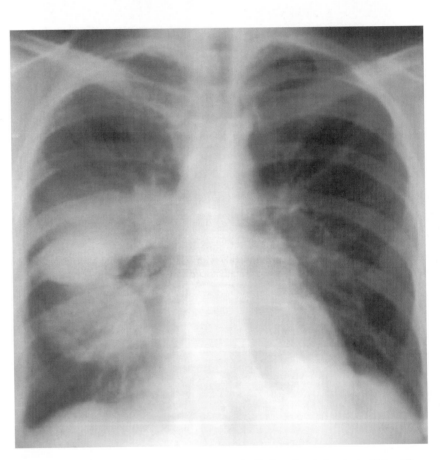

**FIGURE 2-26.** CXR depicting a loculated pleural effusion that is located within a fissure that is sometimes mistaken for a tumor and thus is called a pseudotumor or phantom tumor.

**HIGH-YIELD FACTS**

**Chest Radiology**

## Empyema (Fig. 2-27)

### CAUSE

Inflammatory fluid within the pleural space most commonly due to infectious causes (60%). The remaining causes include trauma and postsurgical.

### CHEST X-RAY FINDINGS

- Often elliptical in shape and loculated.
- May contain air, which is most often due to a bronchopleura "bronchopleural" fistula.
- It does not move freely or layer on a decubitus x-ray.

A chest CT is the best way to further characterize and locate an empyema for possible drainage.

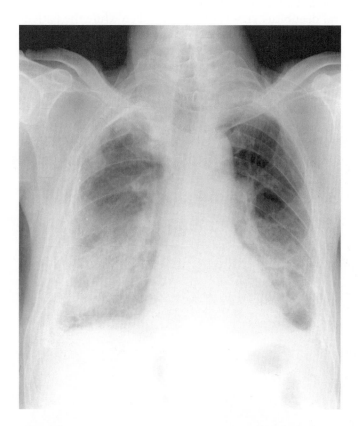

FIGURE 2-27. **CXR in a patient with empyema showing markedly thickened pleura bilaterally with calcified pleural plaques and resultant volume loss.**

■ Deep sulcus sign: A deep lateral costophrenic angle seen on the supine view.

■ Tension PTX is an emergency!

■ Expiratory and/or decubitus views are other views to verify if a PTX is present.

### Pneumothorax (PTX) (Fig. 2-28)

#### CAUSE

Due to air entering the "pleural" space, most commonly due to trauma.

#### CHEST X-RAY FINDINGS

■ Simple PTX: Very thin white line (visceral pleura), with no lung marking beyond that line.
■ Tension PTX: The above findings with a contralateral mediastinal shift. The involved hemithorax is dark and expanded.
■ On a supine view the only sign of a PTX maybe the *deep sulcus* sign.
■ **Expiration view**: Patient exhales as x-ray is taken. The lung will retract, and the visceral line will be accentuated at the apex of the lung. This will confirm a pneumothorax.
■ **Lateral decubitus view**: An x-ray is taken while the patient is lying laterally on the opposite side of the suspected pneumothorax. For example, if a right pneumothorax is suspected, the patient will lie on his left side. Air will rise to the top and accentuate the visceral pleural line.

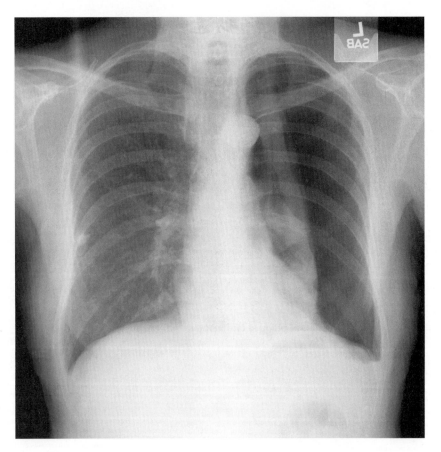

**FIGURE 2-28. CXR demonstrates left-sided pneumothorax. Note the complete lack of lung markings.**

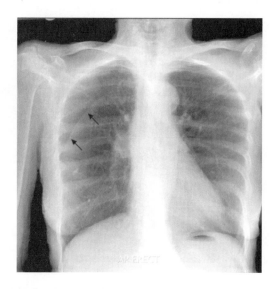

**FIGURE 2-29.** **CXR depicting skin fold (arrows) which can mimic a pneumothorax.**

Notice thickness of the line and lung markings beyond the line. (Reproduced, with permission, *Imaging* 18: 111–121. © 2006, The British Institute of Radiology.)

## Skin Fold (Fig. 2-29)

### CAUSE

A normal skin edge, which you may see on a chest x-ray.

### CHEST X-RAY FINDINGS

- Look for a thick line (as opposed to a thin line with a PTX).
- Look for lung markings beyond the thick line (a PTX would have no lung markings beyond the visceral pleura line).

## Pneumomediastinum (Fig. 2-30)

### CAUSES

Esophageal injury, tracheobronchial tear, respiratory illness such as obstructive lung disease, or elevated alveolar pressures, which can be due to forceful coughing, Valsalva maneuver, etc.

### CHEST X-RAY FINDINGS

- Usually linear collections of air in the upper mediastinum
- On the lateral view there may be air outlying the trachea.

If you are uncertain if it is a PTX or skin fold, an expiration or decubitus view can be ordered to differentiate between the two.

Pneumomediastium:
- May be associated with a PTX.
- Suspect in trauma patient who has a persistent collection of air despite a chest tube.

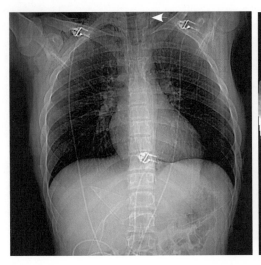
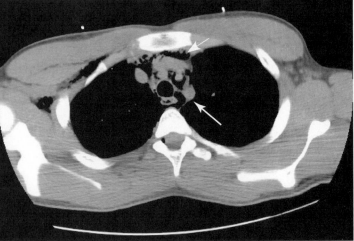

**FIGURE 2-30.** Scout view on the left depicting lucency along left mediastinal border (arrow) indicating pneumomediastinum.

Also note the subcutaneous emphysema on the right side (arrowhead). CT on the right confirms subcutaneous emphysema (arrowhead) and extensive pneumomediastinum (arrow).

- Seventy percent of mesotheliomas are associated with asbestos exposure.

### Pleural Calcification (Fig. 2-31)

#### CAUSE

Most likely due to an old calcified empyema or asbestosis.

#### CHEST X-RAY FINDINGS

- Old empyema: Usually unilateral calcifications along the pleura
- Asbestosis: Usually bilateral pleural calcification

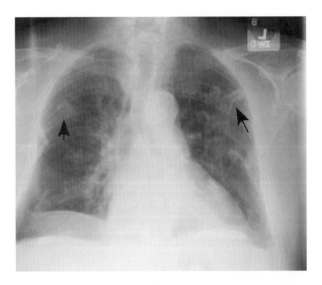

**FIGURE 2-31.** CXR depicting multiple calcified pleural plaques consistent with asbestosis exposure.

## Aortic Dissection (Fig. 2-32)

### CAUSES

Due to an intimal tear. Hypertension is the most common cause. Increased incidence in patients with Marfan's, coarctation of the aorta, and bicuspid aortic valve.

### IMAGING FINDINGS

- Chest x-ray: Be suspicious if there is a dilated aorta, widened mediastinum, and cardiomegaly.
- CT: The key finding is identification of a double lumen, representing the true and false lumina.

Stanford type A dissection involves the ascending "and +/– descending aortas." Stanford B dissection involves only the descending aorta. Type A requires surgery for treatment. Type B is treated medically.

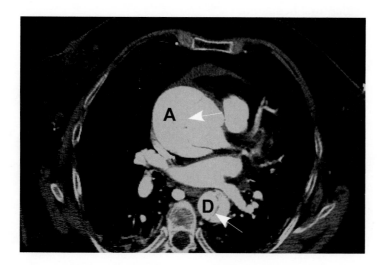

**FIGURE 2-32. Chest CT demonstrating type A Stanford aortic dissection.**

Note presence of the flap (arrow) in the ascending aorta (A) as well as the descending aorta (D).

Aortic Transection:
- A dissection and a transection are not the same thing!
- On chest x-ray, mediastinal widening is the most sensitive diagnostic sign, but if it is the only sign, the specificity is only 10%.
- If there is an uncertainty of an abnormality on the CT scan, transcatheter aortography should be performed.

### Aortic Transection (Fig. 2-33)

#### CAUSES

Due to rapid deceleration injuries. Usually, the tear is located just distal to the origin of the left subclavian artery at the aortic isthmus.

#### IMAGING FINDINGS

- Chest x-ray:
  - Mediastinal widening greater than 8 cm
  - Obscured aortic knob
  - Abnormal paraspinous stripes
  - Blood in the apex of the lung, known as the *apical cap sign*
  - NG tube, trachea, or endotracheal tube deviated to the right
- CT:
  - Aortic pseudoaneurysm
  - Aortic intraluminal filling defect
  - Abnormal aortic contour
  - Mediastinal hematoma

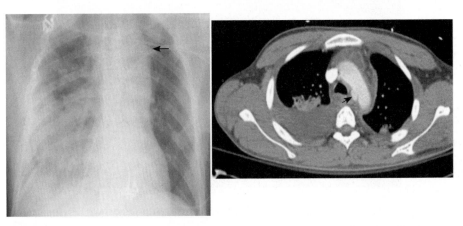

FIGURE 2-33. **CXR demonstrates indeterminate aortic knob and widened mediastinum (arrow). CT on right from the same patient shows acute aortic transection with a pseudoaneurysm formation (arrow) and surrounding mediastinal hematoma (arrow).**

## Thoracic Aortic Aneurysms (Fig. 2-34)

### CAUSES

- Atherosclerotic
- Traumatic
- Congenital
- Cystic medial necrosis
- Inflammatory

### IMAGING FINDINGS

- Chest x-ray: Widening of the ascending aorta or aortic arch
- CT: A CT with IV contrast is usually ordered for further evaluation to see the lumen as well as the amount of clot along the inner wall. Enlargement of the aorta greater than 5 cm is considered an aneurysm.

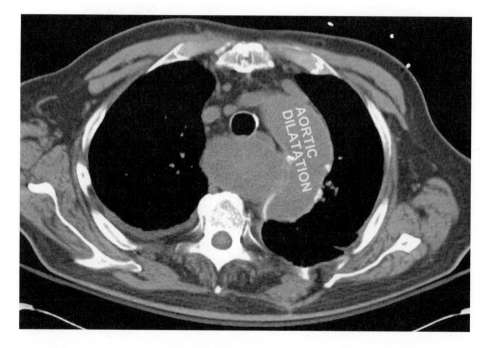

**FIGURE 2-34. Chest CT demonstrating gross aneurysmal dilatation of the aorta.**

## Pulmonary Embolus (Fig. 2-35)

### CAUSES

Hypercoagulable states, recent surgery or pregnancy, prolonged immobilization, or underlying malignancy.

### IMAGING FINDINGS

- Chest x-ray:
  - Initially usually normal.
  - May progress to show atelectasis, small pleural effusion, and an elevated hemidiaphragm.
  - Later, if the embolism results in infarction, a wedge-shaped opacity in the periphery of the lung known as a *Hampton hump* may be seen.
- CT: Central filling defect(s) within the main, segmental, or subsegmental pulmonary arteries.

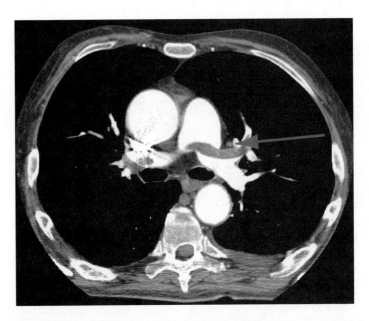

**FIGURE 2-35. Chest CT demonstrating pulmonary embolism.**

Filling defect (arrow).

## Pulmonary Hypertension

### CAUSES

ASD, VSD, PDA, pulmonary emboli, COPD, mitral valve disease, left ventricular failure, lung disease

### IMAGING FINDINGS

Enlargement of both the left and right pulmonary arteries with attenuation of the peripheral vessels (Fig. 2-36).

The treatment of pulmonary hypertension is primarily directed at treatment of the underlying disease.

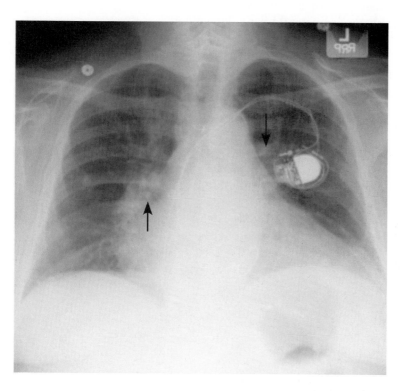

**FIGURE 2-36.** CXR depicting enlargement of the central pulmonary arteries (arrows) suggestive of pulmonary artery hypertension.

Sarcoidosis is most prevalent in the African-American female population.

- Sarcoid has bilateral LN enlargement, and non-caseating granulomas. TB has unilateral LN enlargement and caseating granulomas.
- Cavitation is the hallmark of post–primary infection, and indicates transmissible disease.

**HIGH-YIELD FACTS**

**Chest Radiology**

### Sarcoidosis (Fig. 2-37)

#### CAUSE

Unknown etiology. Characterized by noncaseating epithelioid granulomas that may affect any organ system.

#### IMAGING FINDINGS

Chest x-ray and chest CT:

- Stage 0: Normal chest radiograph
  - Stage 1: Bilateral hilar enlargement
  - Stage 2: Bilateral hilar enlargement and lung infiltrates
  - Stage 3: Pulmonary infiltrates
  - Stage 4: Pulmonary fibrosis

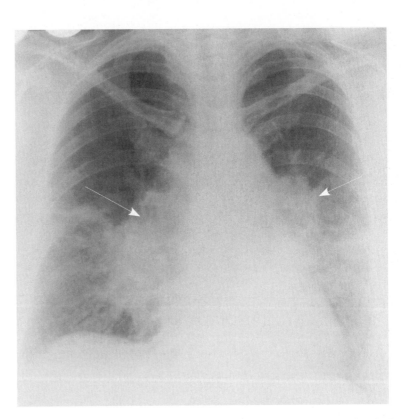

**FIGURE 2-37. CXR demonstrates bilateral massive hilar (arrows) and mediastinal adenopathy with infiltrates in both midlung fields, consistent with sarcoidosis.**

## CAUSE

Caused by *Mycobacterium tuberculosis*

## IMAGING FINDINGS

- **Primary TB:** Focal middle or lower lobe infiltrate with hilar lymph node (LN) enlargement
- **Reactivation TB:** Occurs in the upper lobes and superior segment of the lower lobe. Nodular opacities are usually seen. This can progress to cavitations, empyema, and miliary TB (Fig. 2-38).
- **Miliary TB:** Multiple tiny nodules are diffusely spread throughout the lung. This can occur during or after the primary or reactivation stage.

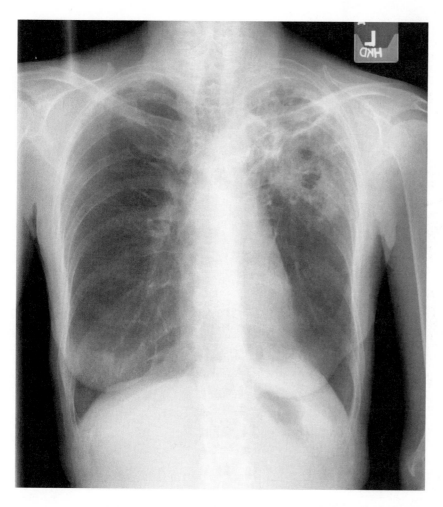

**FIGURE 2-38.** Cavitary mass in the LUL with volume losss. Active TB cannot be excluded.

### Endotracheal Tube (Fig. 2-39)

- Ideal location: Tip should be 2-6 cm above the carina.
- Misplaced tube: Can be placed too high, too low within the esophagus, or mainstem bronchus

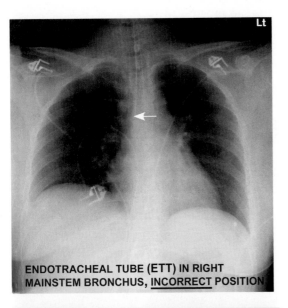

ENDOTRACHEAL TUBE (ETT) IN RIGHT MAINSTEM BRONCHUS, <u>INCORRECT</u> POSITION

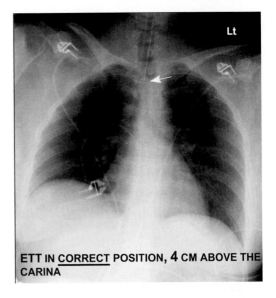

ETT IN <u>CORRECT</u> POSITION, **4** CM ABOVE THE CARINA

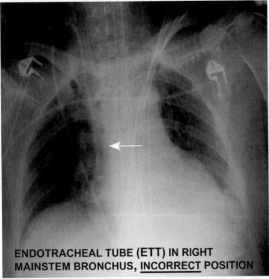

ENDOTRACHEAL TUBE (ETT) IN RIGHT MAINSTEM BRONCHUS, <u>INCORRECT</u> POSITION

**FIGURE 2-39.** Incorrect (2 left panels) and correct (right panel) psitions of endotrachael tube (ETT).

## Chest Tube (Fig. 2-40)

- Ideal location: Tip and side ports are inside the chest cavity.
- Misplaced line: Tube can be kinked or not within the chest cavity.

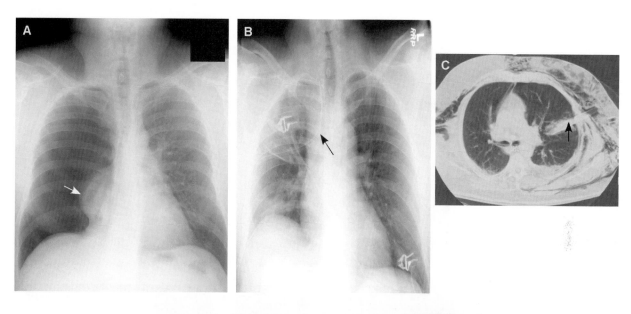

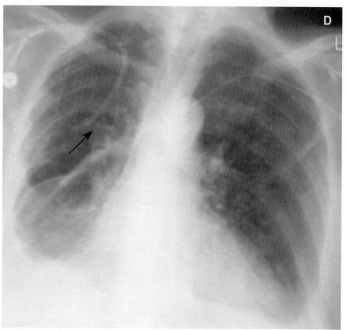

**FIGURE 2-40. Chest tube placement.**

Panel A demonstrates mild tension pneumothorax with mediastinal shift and collapsed lung on the right (white arrow). Panel B is the CXR in the same patient demonstrating resolution of the pneumothorax after placement of single chest tube in correct position (black arrow). Panel C, from a different patient, is a chest CT depicting grossly incorrect placement of chest tube into left lung parenchyma (black arrow). Panel D demonstrates kinked right sided chest tube (arrow).

## Nasogastric Tube (Fig. 2-41)

- Ideal location: Tip within the stomach
- Misplaced tube: Most commonly in the distal esophagus, coiled in the upper esophagus, or within the bronchus

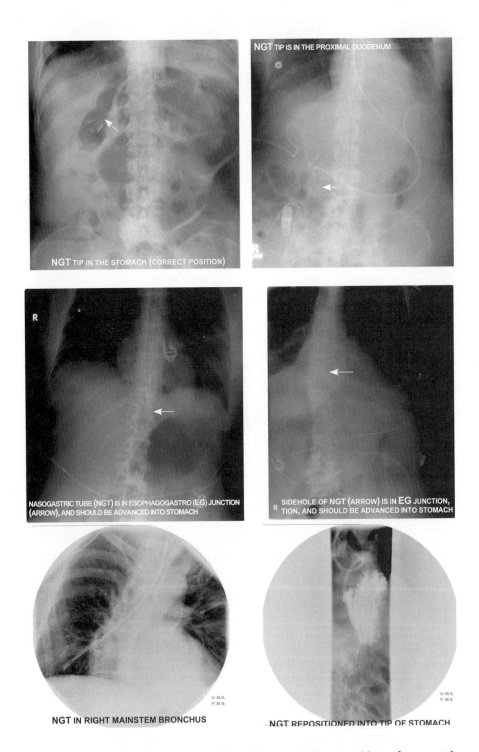

**FIGURE 2-41. Correct (top left and right) and incorrect (others) positions of nasogastric tubes.**

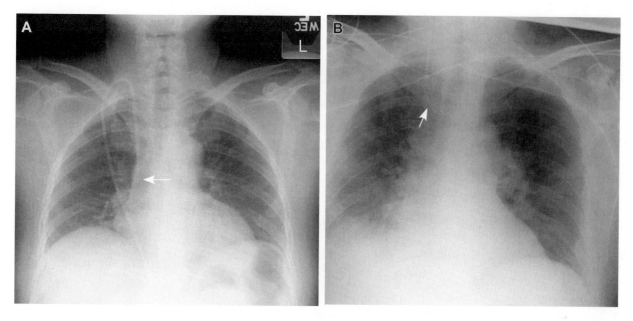

**FIGURE 2-42. Jugular vein catheter placement.**

Panel A shows a CXR depicting correct position of internal jugular vein catheter at the junction of the SVC and the right atrium. Panel B demonstrates incorrect positioning with catheter coiled in the SVC. SVC, superior vena cava.

## Jugular or Subclavian Central Venous Line (Fig. 2-42)

- Ideal location is the cavo-atrial junction.
- Misplaced line can turn up the internal jugular vein, right atrium, or coiled in the superior vena cava (SVC).

## Pulmonary Artery Catheter (Swan-Ganz Catheter) (Fig. 2-43)

- Ideal location: Proximal pulmonary artery
- Misplaced line: If inserted too far into the pulmonary artery, an infarct can occur

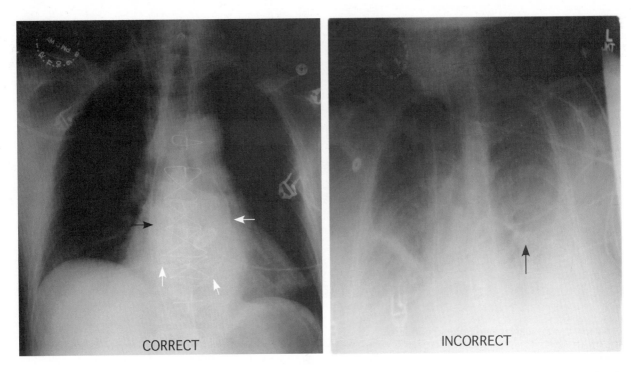

CORRECT          INCORRECT

FIGURE 2-43. CXR demonstrating correct (left panel) and incorrect (right panel) positioning of pulmonary artery catheter.

## Umbilical Vein Catheter (Fig. 2-44)

- Ideal location: Level of T9 vertebra, at the junction of inferior vena cava and right atrium
- Misplaced line can turn up in the right portal vein

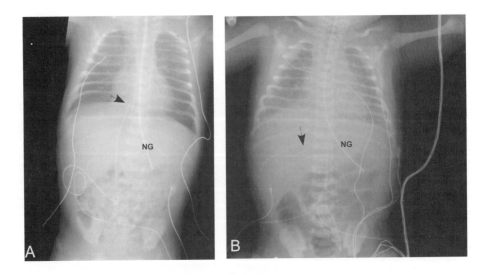

FIGURE 2-44. Umbilical vein in correct (A) and incorrect (B) positions.

## Cardiac Pacemaker (Fig. 2-45)

- Ideal location: Tips within the right atrium and right ventricle

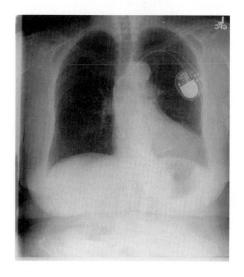 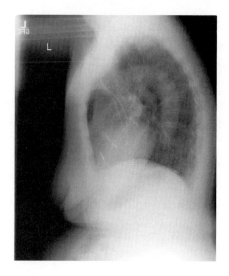

**FIGURE 2-45. Cardiac pacemaker.**

### ▶ REVIEW OF EMERGENCY FINDINGS

- Tension pneumothorax (see Fig. 2-46)
- Supine pneumothorax (see Fig. 2-47)
- Free air under the diaphragm (see Fig. 2-48)
- Pneumomediastinum (see Fig. 2-30)
- Aortic dissection (see Fig. 2-32)
- Aortic injury (see Fig. 2-33)
- Feeding tube in bronchus (see Fig. 2-41)

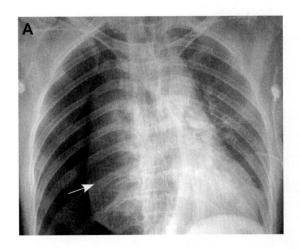

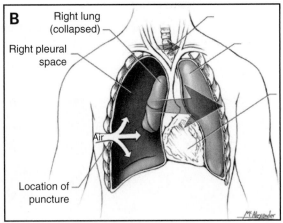

**FIGURE 2-46. Tension pneumothorax.**

(A) CXR demonstrating tension pneumothorax. Note right collapsed lung (arrow). This is a life threatening diagnosis that should be made clinically, rather than delaying to obtain a radiograph. (Reproduced, with permission, from McRoberts R., et al.: Emerg Med J 2005;22:597–598, BMJ Publishing Group Ltd.) (B) Schematic of tension pneumothorax.

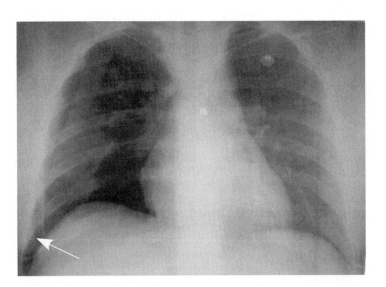

**FIGURE 2-47. Chest x-ray demonstrates a large right pneumothorax with widening and deepening of the right costophrenic angle, also known as the deep sulcus sign (arrow).**

Occasionally, this sign is the only radiographic indication of a pneumothorax in a supine patient. (Reproduced, with permission, from Stone CK, Humphries RL: *Current Emergency Diagnosis and Treatment*, 6th ed., McGraw-Hill, 2008: 348.)

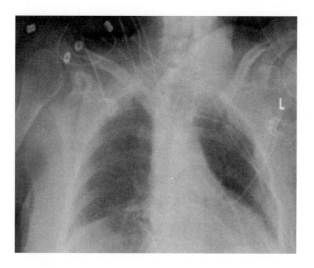

**FIGURE 2-48.** CXR depicting lucency under the right hemidiaphragm consistent with free intraperitoneal air.

# HIGH-YIELD FACTS IN

# Gastrointestinal Radiology

- Plain abdominal film
- Ultrasound
- Intraluminal contrast studies
- CT scan
- MRI
- CT angiogram
- CT enterography
- MR angiogram
- Conventional angiogram
- Endoscopic studies
- Nuclear imaging
- Percutaneous imaging procedures

## Plain Abdominal Film

Often the first preliminary test

### INDICATIONS

- Bowel obstruction
- Viscus perforation
- Foreign body ingestion

### ADVANTAGES

- Easy availability
- Low cost

### LIMITATIONS

- Screening modality; usually need another imaging test to confirm diagnosis
- Lack of anatomic detail

### HOW TO READ AN ABDOMINAL FILM

See Figure 3-1.

- Make sure the film belongs to the right patient.
- Identify the sides correctly and inspect the liver and spleen shadows.
- Bilateral renal outlines should be present and symmetric and smooth. Right kidney is lower than left.
- Bilateral psoas shadows should be symmetric.
- Urinary bladder may or may not be outlined depending on the degree of distention.
- Visualized bony structures should be inspected for abnormality.
- Identify normal bowel gas pattern.

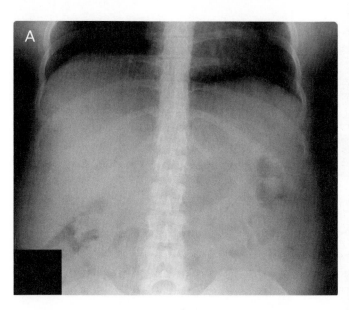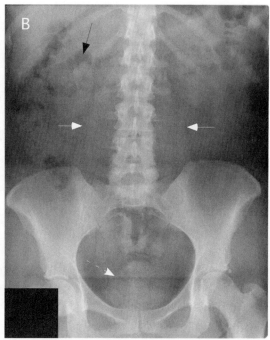

**FIGURE 3-1. Normal kidney, ureter, and bladder (KUB).**

(A) Top half with domes of the diaphragm. (B) Lower half of the abdomen. Note psoas shadows (white arrows), urinary bladder (broken arrow), and bowel gas (black arrow).

## Abdominal Ultrasound (Fig. 3-2)

### APPROACHES

- Superficial
- Endoscopic: Assisting probes are used in upper GI, pancreaticobiliary, and colorectal pathologies for staging malignancies

### INDICATIONS

- Gallbladder and hepatic pathology
- Delineation and differentiation of intra-abdominal cystic structures
- Trauma; FAST (focused abdominal sonography in trauma) is a very useful tool in assessment of trauma patients
- Emerging role of endoscopic ultrasound in biliary and pancreatic pathologies
- Guiding procedures
- Doppler studies for evaluation of vascular structures

### ADVANTAGES

Inexpensive, noninvasive, no contrast

### LIMITATIONS

- Operator dependent
- Inferior for assessment of bowel pathology due to artifact from air
- Lack of mucosal detail

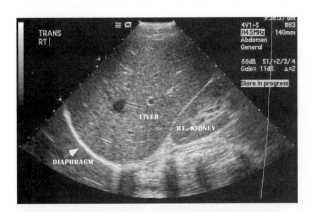
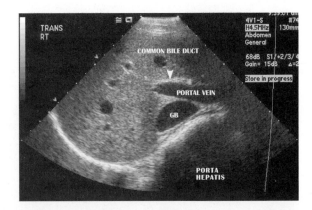
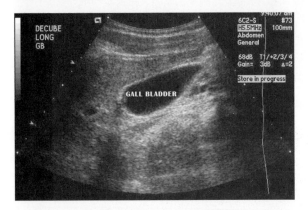
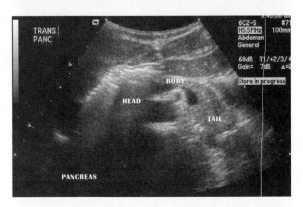
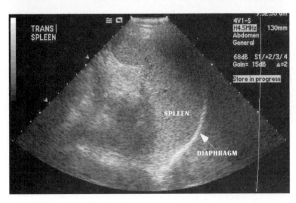
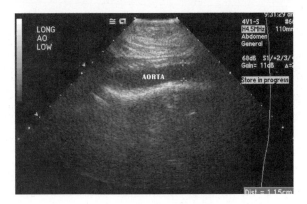

**FIGURE 3-2. Normal abdominal ultrasound.**

### Abdominal CT (Fig. 3-3)

#### *INDICATIONS*

- Assessment of acute abdomen and to rule out conditions such as acute appendicitis, acute pancreatitis, small bowel obstruction, colitis.
- Trauma
- CT angiograms for suspected vascular leaks, aneurysm, bowel infarctions
- CT enterography is being used for inflammatory bowel diseases (Crohn's disease).
- Virtual CT colonoscopy: Not yet a very widely used tool

#### *ADVANTAGES*

Excellent cross-sectional imaging modality that provides functional information as well

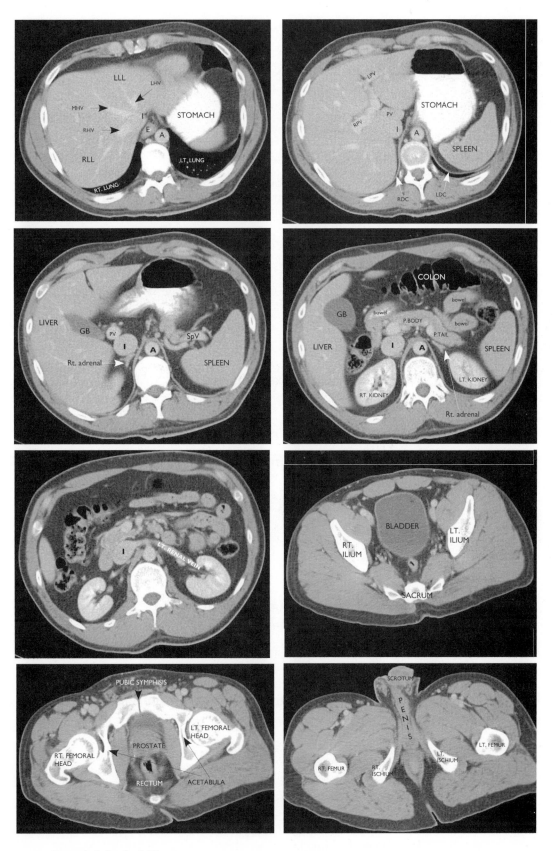

**FIGURE 3-3. Normal abdominal CT.**

Rt, right; Lt, left; LLL, left lobe of liver; RLL, right lobe of liver; RHV, right hepatic vein; MHV, middle hepatic vein; LHV, left hepatic vein; I, inferior vena cava; A, aorta; E, esophagus; LPV, left portal vein; RPV, right portal vein; PV, portal vein; RDC, right diaphragm crus; LDC, left diaphragm crus; spv, splenic vein; GB, gallbladder; P. Body, body of pancreas; P. Tail, tail of pancreas; SpV, splenic vein.

- Availability
- Radiation exposure
- Expensive

## MRI

### ADVANTAGES

- Superior soft tissue detail
- Excellent cross-sectional imaging tool for evaluation and staging of malignancies, especially rectal and esophageal, inflammatory and obstructive pathologies

### DISADVANTAGES

- Higher cost
- Contraindicated in patients with metallic hardware
- Long imaging time
- Claustrophobia

## Intraluminal Contrast Examinations

### CONTRAST MEDIA

- Barium and iodine containing water soluble contrast medium (iodograffin).
- The latter is used in evaluation of suspected perforated viscus.

## Barium Swallow (Figs. 3-4 through 3-7)

### INDICATION

Esophageal pathologies

## Single- or Double-Contrast Upper GI Series

### INDICATIONS

Imaging of pharynx, esophagus, stomach, and duodenum

## Small Bowel Follow-Through Examination and Enteroclysis

### INDICATIONS

Imaging of small intestinal and ileocecal pathologies

## Single- or Double-Contrast Enemas

### INDICATIONS

Imaging of the large intestine

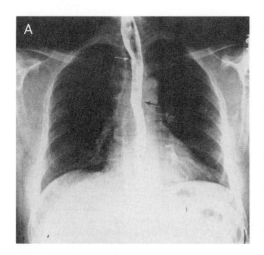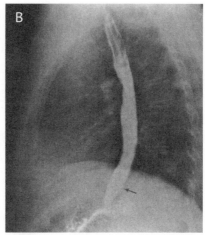

**FIGURE 3-4. Barium esophagogram.**

(A) Posteroanterior view. (B) Lateral view. White arrow shows deviation to the left; black arrow shows return to midline. Black arrow on lateral view shows anterior deviation. (Reproduced, with permission, from Rothberg M, DeMeester TR: Surgical anatomy of the esophagus. In Shields TW (ed.): *General Thoracic Surgery*, 3rd ed. Philadelphia: Lea & Febiger, 1989: 77.)

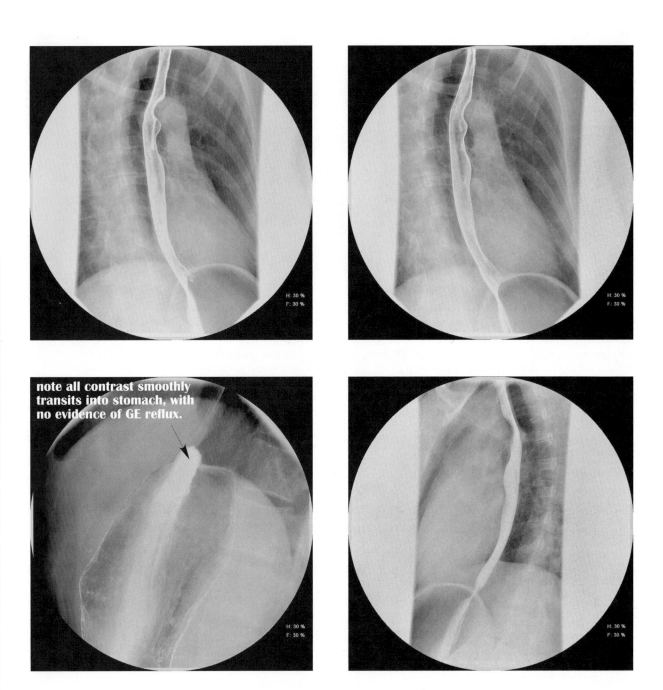

note all contrast smoothly transits into stomach, with no evidence of GE reflux.

**FIGURE 3-5.** Video esophagogram demonstrating normal swallowing and peristalsis through the esophagus.

No evidence of any gastroesophageal reflux.

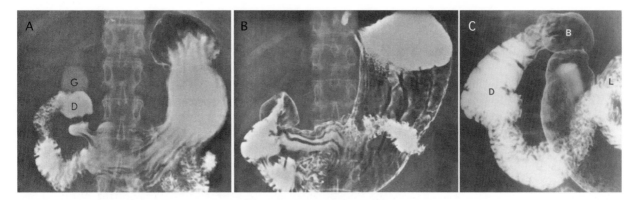

**FIGURE 3-6. Upper GI series.**

(A) Prone frontal radiograph of stomach and duodenum from a single-contrast upper GI examination. The duodenal bulb (D) is attached to the gastric antrum by the pyloric channel. The gallbladder (G) is also opacified from an oral cholecystogram. (B) Supine frontal film of the stomach and duodenum from a double-contrast upper GI examination in which a high-density barium suspension and gas crystals ($CO_2$) are used. Compared to A, the stomach is better distended primarily by the generated gas. (C) Radiograph of the duodenum showing the duodenal bulb (B) attached to the gastric antrum. The descending duodenum (D) extends from the apex of the bulb to the inferior duodenal flexure. The horizontal and ascending portions of the duodenum terminate at the duodenojejunal junction (L), which is attached to the ligament of Treitz. (Reproduced, with permission, from Chen MY, Pope TL, Ott DJ: *Basic Radiology*. New York: McGraw-Hill, 2004: 247, 248, 250.)

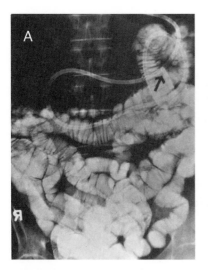
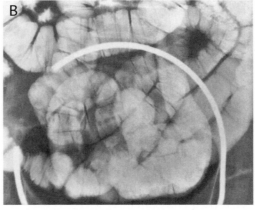

**FIGURE 3-7. Enteroclysis.**

(A) Large film of the abdomen from an enteroclysis examination of the small intestine. The small bowel is intubated with the tip of the tube (arrow) in the jejunum. Compared to the perioral examination, the small bowel loops are distended more fully, causing the mucosal folds to assume a transverse orientation. (B) Compression film (ring of balloon paddle) of the small bowel loops in the pelvis with the patient in a prone position. Although the loops are overlapped, the "see-through" effect using a dilute barium suspension permits their clear visualization. (Reproduced, with permission, from Chen MY, Pope TL, Ott DJ: *Basic Radiology*. New York: McGraw-Hill, 2004: 251.)

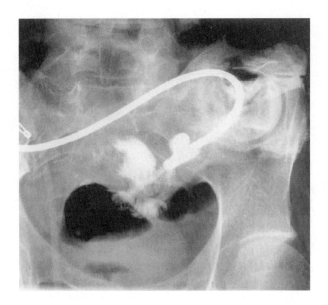

**FIGURE 3-8. Fistulogram.**

Contrast injected into a catheter placed into the fistula tract demonstrates communication with the small intestine in this patient with Crohn's disease. (Reproduced, with permission, from Brunicardi FC, Andersen DK, Billiar TR, et al.: *Schwartz's Principles of Surgery*, 8th ed. New York: McGraw-Hill, 2005: 1038.)

## Fistulograms and Sinograms (Fig. 3-8)

### *INDICATIONS*

May be used in postoperative patients for assessment of fistulae and sinus tracts

## Endoscopy

### *INDICATIONS*

- Upper and lower GI endoscopy enable direct visualization and directed biopsies.
- Endoscopic retrograde cholangiopancreaticography (ERCP) visualizes the hepatobiliary tree.

## ERCP (Fig. 3-9)

Involves introduction of an endoscope into the duodenum followed by cannulation of the biliary tree. It is often performed along with papillotomy, which serves as a therapeutic intervention for biliary calculi and drainage procedures of obstructed bile ducts.

### INDICATIONS

- Diagnostic ERCP is indicated in jaundice of unclear origin and suspected pancreatic disease such as chronic pancreatitis and pseudocysts.
- Primary approach for drainage and stenting of benign and malignant biliary obstruction, the main advantage being that the liver need not be punctured.
- If the papilla cannot be cannulated or the obstruction cannot be passed with a guidewire, a percutaneous transhepatic approach may be tried. However, in difficult and postoperative cases, noninvasive methods such as magnetic resonance cholangiopancreatography (MRCP) are increasingly being used for evaluation.

### COMPLICATIONS

Pancreatitis, duodenal perforation, duodenal hemorrhage, hepatic and splenic injury, infection, and stent misplacement

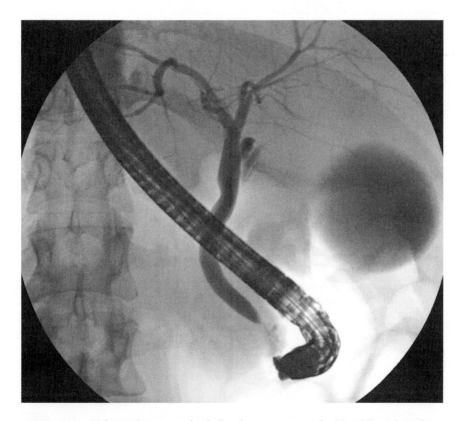

**FIGURE 3-9.** Endoscopic retrograde cholangiopancreatography (ERCP) is an invasive technique used to demonstrate the anatomy of the biliary tree and pancreatic duct through contrast opacification of the ductal system.

### LOCATION AND CAUSE (FIG. 3-10)

Neuronal degeneration within the Auerbach's plexus in the esophagus

### TYPES

Primary or secondary (scleroderma)

### IMAGING

Barium swallow reveals dilated esophagus with distal tapering and narrowing.

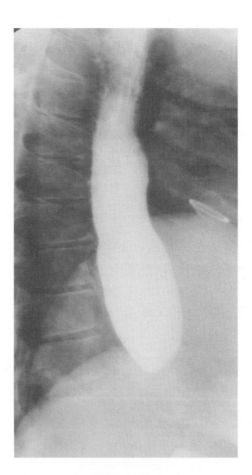

FIGURE 3-10. **Barium esophagogram in a patient with achalasia demonstrates a dilated esophagus with a sharply tapered "bird beak" narrowing.**

Most common esophageal diverticulum

### CAUSE

A pulsion diverticulum caused by increased intraluminal pressure

### LOCATION

Outpouching of pharyngeal mucosa above the cricopharyngeus (upper esophageal sphincter)

### IMAGING

Diagnosis can be made by barium esophagogram or endoscopy. Barium esophagogram reveals a barium-filled outpouching in the region of the esophageal inlet.

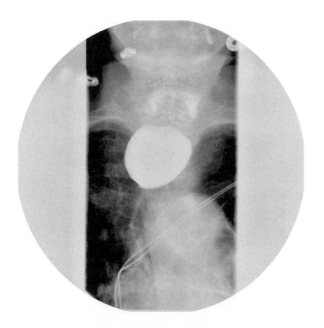 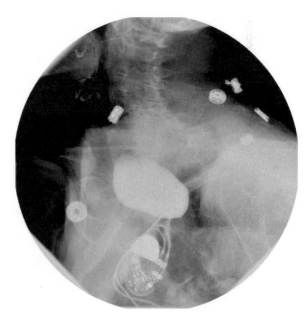

FIGURE 3-11. Zenker's diverticulum.

### CAUSE

Ulcer, gastritis, vascular malformation

### LOCATION

Stomach and duodenum

### IMAGING

- Upper GI endoscopy is the definitive test for diagnosis and appropriate intervention.
- Barium upper GI series may be done if endoscopy is unavailable and may reveal collection of contrast within the ulcer crater. Gastritis and duodenitis are manifested by thickened folds.
- Other tests for further investigation include radionuclide studies and angiography.

► **SMALL BOWEL OBSTRUCTION (FIG. 3-12)**

### CAUSES

- Extrinsic: Hernias, adhesions, masses, volvulus
- Intrinsic: Gallstones, foreign bodies

### LOCATION

- Small bowel loops are centrally located as compared to the large bowel.
- Valvulae conniventes are thinner than the colonic haustral folds.

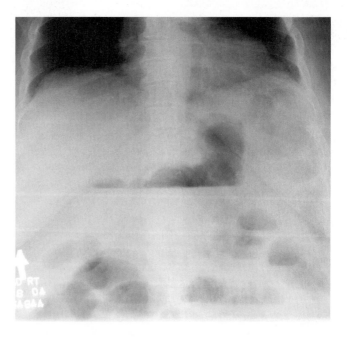

**FIGURE 3-12.** Radiograph of the abdomen demonstrates multiple distended centrally located small bowel loops with air-fluid levels throughout the abdomen.

## IMAGING

- **Plain x-ray:**
  - First preliminary investigation
  - **Advantages:** Usually helpful in establishing diagnosis. In rare cases, may be able to define the point of transition.
  - **Disadvantages:** Difficult to ascertain definitive etiology. Plain films are diagnostic in 50% to 60%, equivocal in 20% to 30%, and misleading in 10% to 20% of cases.
- **CT:**
  - **Advantages:** Clear diagnosis in equivocal cases, detailed anatomy with definitive cause and point of transition, differentiating paralytic ileus from anatomic obstruction
- **Goals of imaging:**
  - **Establish a diagnosis:** Air fluid levels, dilated bowel loops
  - **Complete vs. incomplete:** No bowel gas beyond the level of obstruction in a complete obstruction

## COMPLICATIONS

Strangulation, perforation (Fig. 3-13)

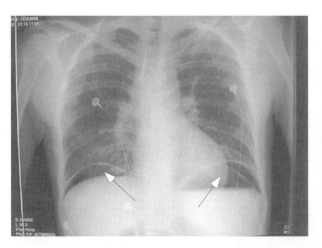 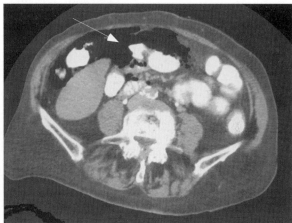

**FIGURE 3-13.** Plain film and CT demonstrating free air under the diaphragm secondary to perforation of small bowel.

► **COLONIC OBSTRUCTION (FIG. 3-14)**

Hypaque enema may be therapeutic in large bowel obstruction.

### CAUSE

Hernias, adhesions, masses, volvulus

### LOCATION

Peripherally located dilated bowel loops with haustral folds

### IMAGING

Plain x-ray for initial diagnosis. CT to confirm diagnosis and ascertain underlying cause. In large bowel obstruction, hypaque enema may be diagnostic as well as therapeutic.

► **COLITIS**

**Types**: Ulcerative colitis and Crohn's disease

### Infectious Colitis (Fig. 3-15)

- C. *difficile* is a common cause.
- Seen in patients on antimicrobial treatment.

### LOCATION

- Can affect ascending, transverse, and descending colon.

### IMAGING

- CT scan is the investigation of choice and reveals colonic wall thickening. See Figure 3-16.
- Plain x-ray may reveal bowel wall thickening or proximal bowel obstruction.

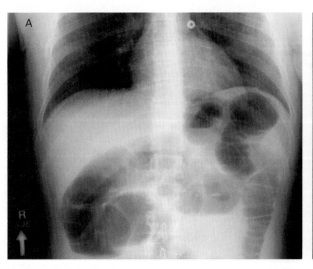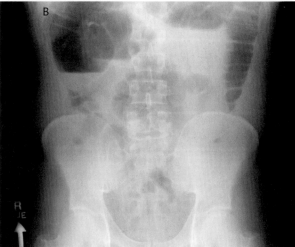

**FIGURE 3-14. Supine (A) and erect (B) films demonstrating a dilated colon.**

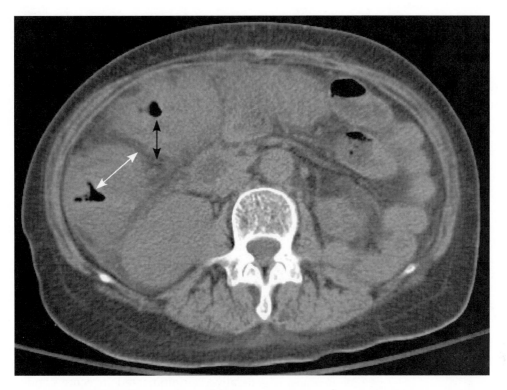

FIGURE 3-15. CT demonstrating marked wall thickening in the ascending colon (white arrow) and the transverse colon (black arrow) in a patient with *C. difficile* colitis.

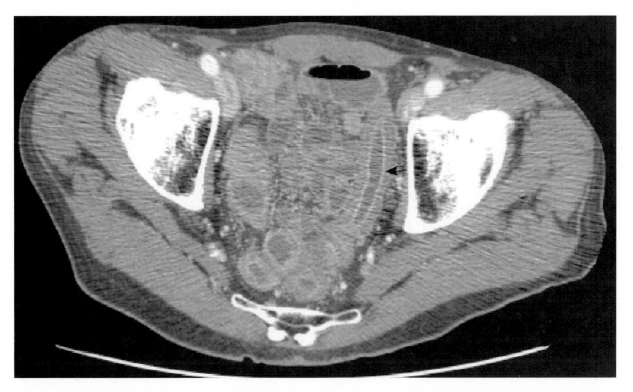

FIGURE 3-16. CT enterography depicting thickening of the sigmoid colon (arrow) in a patient with ulcerative colitis.

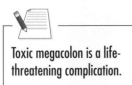
### COMPLICATIONS

- Toxic megacolon
- Perforation

## Inflammatory Colitis

- Include ulcerative colitis and Crohn's disease

## Ulcerative Colitis (Fig. 3-16)

### LOCATION

Primarily involves large bowel. Rectal involvement with variable contiguous, proximal involvement is most common.

### IMAGING

- Plain radiography can readily detect toxic megacolon, one of the serious complications.
- Double-contrast barium enema can readily detect mucosal changes of ulcerative colitis, namely, mucosal thickening, irregularity, and superficial ulceration.
- Colonoscopy is generally contraindicated in acute conditions, but is useful for direct visualization and obtaining specimen for histopathologic correlation.
- CT findings are nonspecific and include bowel wall thickening.

## Crohn's Disease (Fig. 3-17)

### *LOCATION*

Most common site of involvement is terminal ileum; can affect any part of GI tract, including the colon.

### *IMAGING*

Intraluminal contrast studies like small bowel follow-through, enteroclysis, and CT enterography are pivotal in establishing diagnosis.

- Barium enema

### *FINDINGS*

Mucosal inflammation with transmural penetration, ulcerations, strictures, skip lesions, abscess formation. No single test is diagnostic.

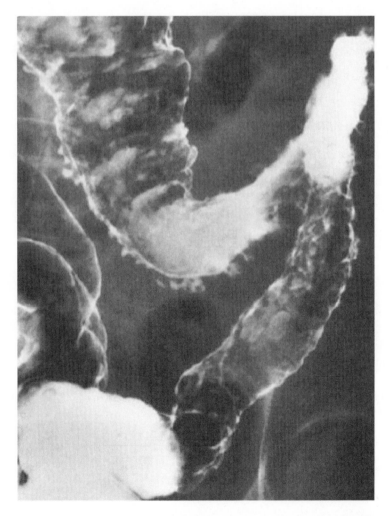

**FIGURE 3-17. Segmental Crohn's disease of the transverse and descending portions of the colon, showing multiple deep ulcers projecting from the margins of the affected colon and small "aphthoid" ulcers appearing like erosions seen in the upper gastrointestinal tract.**

(Reproduced, with permission, from Chen MYM , Pope J, Ott DJ: *Basic Radiology.* accessmedicine.com, McGraw-Hill, 2008.)

### Ischemic Colitis (Fig. 3-18)

**CAUSE**

Compromised blood supply to the colon.

**IMAGING**

- Plain x-ray: Normal or may reveal pneumatosis in the bowel wall or bowel distention.
- CT scan with oral and intravenous contrast may be normal in early cases. Findings are usually nonspecific and include bowel wall thickening. Occasionally, gas may be seen within the mesenteric vein.

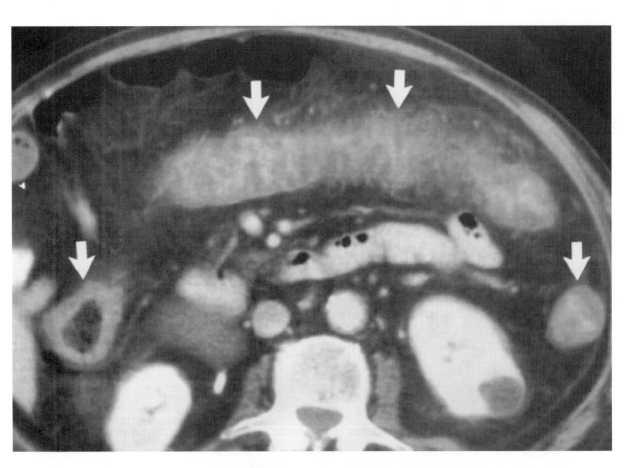

**FIGURE 3-18.** Contrast-enhanced CT scan shows heterogeneous enhancement and wall thickening of the transverse colon, as well as the right and left colon (arrows), with loss of haustral markings.

(Reproduced, with permission, from Balthazar, et al.: *Radiology*, 1999 May;211(2):381-8.)

Common in Western countries. Estimated incidence is 30% at > 60 years and at 60% > 80 years.

### LOCATION

Most common site of involvement is sigmoid colon.

### IMAGING

Abdominal CT is the imaging modality of choice. Look for air-filled mucosal outpouchings in the bowel wall. This is compatible with diverticulosis. Diverticulitis is characterized by associated inflammation manifested by pericolonic stranding.

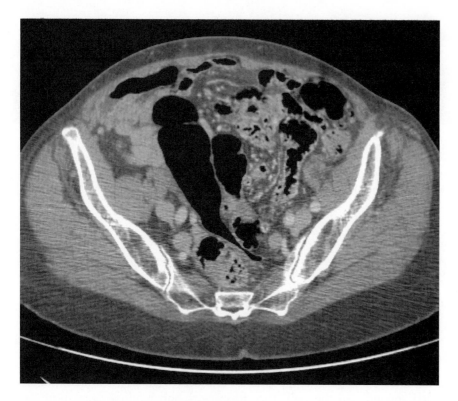

**FIGURE 3-19. CT demonstrating diverticulosis.**

Note small round air- or contrast-filled structures along the colonic lumen. Complications include diverticulitis and hemorrhage.

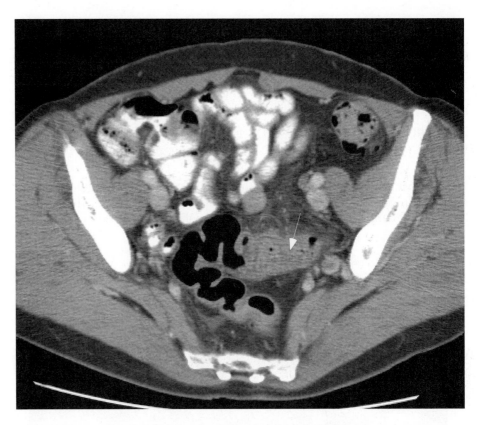

**FIGURE 3-20. Abdominal CT demonstrating sigmoid diverticulitis.**

Note mid-sigmoid thickening with numerous diverticuli and streaking in adjacent pelvic fat. Complications include abscess formation, perforation, strictures, and fistulae.

## ▶ APPENDICITIS (FIG. 3-21)

### *LOCATION*

Right iliac fossa

### *IMAGING*

Abdominal CT is imaging modality of choice. (Fig. 3-21) demonstrates an inflamed appendix in the right iliac fossa, with surrounding streaking in a patient with acute appendicitis.

In pregnant patients, ultrasound or MRI may be used for diagnosis of appendicitis, if clinically indicated.

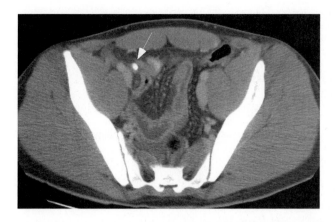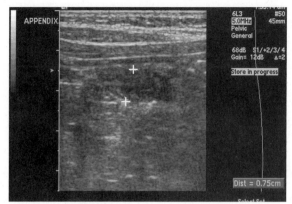

**FIGURE 3-21. Abdominal CT and ultrasound of appendicitis.**

Abdominal CT demonstrates appendicolith (arrow). Findings on ultrasonography suggestive of an inflamed appendix include an outer diameter of > 6 mm, noncompressibility, lack of peristalsis, and periappendiceal fluid collection.

▶ **MIDGUT VOLVULUS (FIG. 3-22)**

- Normally a pediatric condition, caused by nonrotation of the bowel around the superior mesenteric artery.
- Sigmoid and cecal volvulus occur more commonly in adults.

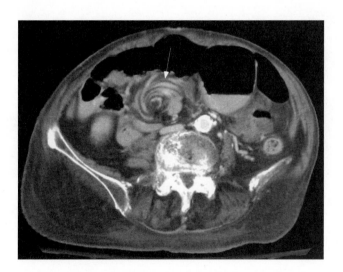

**FIGURE 3-22. CT of the abdomen showing midgut volvulus.**

Arrow points toward the characteristic whirlpool sign, i.e., bowel loops and superior mesenteric vein wrapping around the superior mesenteric artery.

### *LOCATION*

Normal location of the cecum is within the right iliac fossa.

### *CAUSE*

Twisting of the cecum, usually with part of ascending colon along the vertical or transverse axis

### *IMAGING*

- Plain x-ray is usually the first test and is diagnostic. Findings include displaced cecum, small and large bowel obstruction up to the point of torsion, and paucity of gas in the distal colon.
- Hypaque enema (single contrast) may confirm the diagnosis and may also lead to reduction of the volved cecum.
- CT scan reveals the characteristic "swirl sign" as seen in (Fig. 3-23). It is also helpful in delineation of potential complications related to obstruction and vascular compromise.

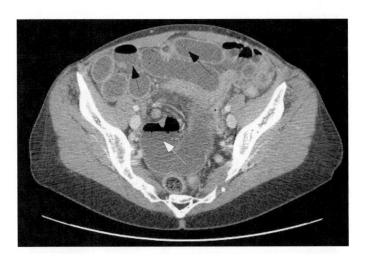

**FIGURE 3-23. CT scan demonstrating cecal volvulus.**

Note the twisted and dilated cecum (white arrow) within the right pelvic cavity. Also note proximally dilated bowel loops (black arrows).

### LOCATION

Normal location of sigmoid colon is in the left lower quadrant.

### CAUSE

Twisting of the sigmoid around its mesenteric axis. Usually in elderly debilitated patients with chronic constipation.

### IMAGING

- Abdominal x-ray is usually diagnostic. It classically reveals double loop (pelvic colon) obstruction with varying degrees of proximal small bowel obstruction. The twisted dilated loop is located in the right side of the abdomen and forms a central double wall that converges in the right lower quadrant called the "coffee bean" sign.
- Single-contrast barium enema is helpful in diagnosis in equivocal cases and may result in decompression and reduction.
- CT scan is useful for delineating complications like vascular ischemia.

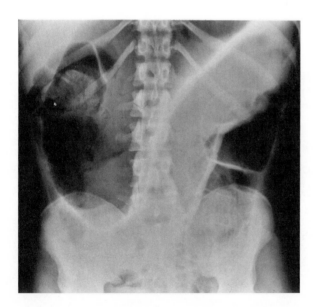

**FIGURE 3-24. AXR shows a grossly distended coffee bean shaped loop of bowel in the right upper quadrant, findings that are typical of a sigmoid volvulus.**

(Reproduced, with permission, from Rozycki GS et al: *Annals of Surgery* (235): 5; May 2002. Lippicott Williams and Wilkins.)

*CAUSES*

- More common in females; seen in 20% of women in the United States, Canada, and Europe.
- Hereditary predisposition.

*IMAGING*

- **Ultrasound:**
  - First-line imaging modality for gallbladder pathologies (Fig. 3-25). demonstrates multiple echogenic (bright) foci within a distended gallbladder with dense distal posterior acoustic dark shadowing (*flashlight sign*) suggestive of gallstones.
  - Always look for associated dilatation and calculi within the biliary ductal system.
  - Limitations of ultrasound include suboptimal visualization of gallbladder due to body habitus, inadequate distention, or overlying bowel gas.
  - Characteristic findings include thickened gallbladder wall, pericholecystic fluid, positive ultrasound, Murphy's sign (tenderness overlying RUQ) (Fig. 3-26).

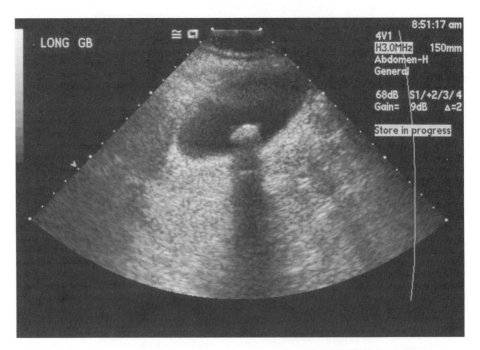

**FIGURE 3-25.** Ultrasound demonstrating gallstone within the gallbladder that produces a bright echo and causes a dark acoustic shadow, giving the characteristic "headlight" appearance.

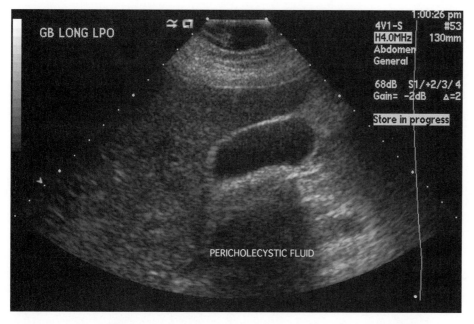

GB LONG LPO

1:00:26 pm
4V1-S          #53
H4.0MHz    130mm
Abdomen
General

68dB   S1/+2/3/ 4
Gain= −2dB    △=2

Store in progress

PERICHOLECYSTIC FLUID

**FIGURE 3-26.** Ultrasound demonstrating acute cholecystitis includes thickened gallbladder wall and pericholecystic fluid.

■ **Hepatobiliary iminodiacetic acid (HIDA) scan (cholescintigraphy) (Fig. 3-27):** May be used in cases where ultrasound is unavailable. Tc-labeled iminodiacetic acid is injected via an IV catheter followed by sequential imaging. Hepatic uptake occurs within the first 15 minutes and the tracer reaches the duodenum in 1 hour. Obstructing gallstones are characterized by lack of uptake of the tracer in the gallbladder and the cystic duct. Gallbladder contraction can be assessed by amount of tracer emptying after administration of cholecystokinin.

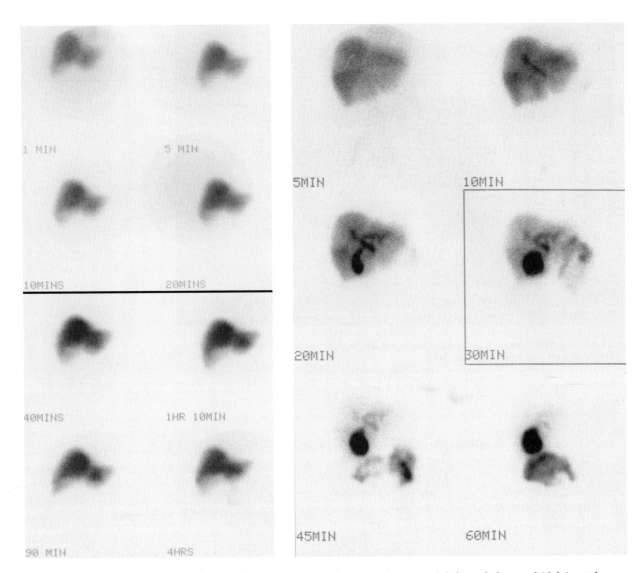

**FIGURE 3-27.** HIDA scan (also known as cholescintigraphy) demonstrating normal (left) and abnormal (right) uptake. The abnormal scan is characteristic of cholecystitis.

### CAUSE

Two most common causes are gallstone disease and alcoholism.

### LOCATION

Pancreas is a retroperitoneal organ.

### IMAGING

- **Plain x-ray**: Not warranted; however, findings may include:
  - The "gasless" abdomen
  - The "sentinel" loop sign, referring to a localized dilated small bowel
  - Prominent air filling and distention of the duodenal loop ("ileus")
  - The "colon cutoff" sign, referring to the abrupt cutoff of the air column within the distended transverse colon at the splenic flexure
  - Pancreatic calcifications, which can be seen with chronic cases
- **CT:**
  - May be equivocal if done 48 hours prior to onset of symptoms.
  - Characteristic findings include bulky, swollen pancreas with surrounding edema; localized fluid collections; abscesses; pancreatic ductal dilatation; and associated complications.
  - There are various scoring systems to grade severity of disease based on CT findings.

> Complications of pancreatitis include:
> - Pleural effusion
> - Pseudocyst
> - Hemorrhage
> - Pseudoaneurysm
> - Splenic vein thrombosis
> - Portal vein thrombosis
> - Superior mesenteric vein thrombosis

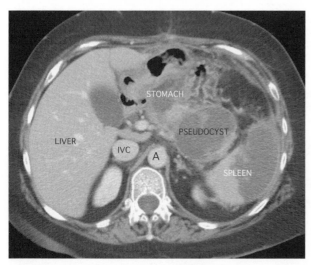

**FIGURE 3-28.** CT of abdomen demonstrates pancreatic pseudocyst with peripancreatic stranding in a patient with pancreatitis.

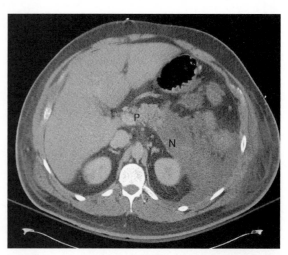

**FIGURE 3.29.** CT of the abodmen demonstrates necrotizing pancreatitis affecting the tail (N) and part of the body of the pancreas. Notice the normal pancreas (P) which does not enhance.

HIGH-YIELD FACTS

Gastrointestinal Radiology

PET utilizes fluorodeoxyglucose (FDG), and is capable of diagnosing malignant involvement of normal-sized nodes that may be missed on other imaging techniques.

Worldwide, esophageal cancer is the 8th most common malignancy.

## ▶ ESOPHAGEAL CANCER (FIG. 3-30)

### TYPES AND LOCATION

- **Squamous cell carcinoma** accounts for 60% and is common in upper esophagus.
- **Adenocarcinoma** usually develops from dysplastic lower esophagus (Barrett's esophagus).

### IMAGING

- Early cancers (limited to mucosa and submucosa with no nodal involvement) may be diagnosed on barium swallow done for evaluation of dysphagia.
- Advanced tumors may appear as a mediastinal mass on plain film, and may cause esophageal dilation with air fluid levels, and achalasia.
- For accurate staging and treatment planning, cross-sectional imaging with CT and endoscopic ultrasound (for depth of involvement) are recommended.
- Positron emission tomography (PET) is increasingly used for more accurate staging due to greater propensity to diagnose metastasis.

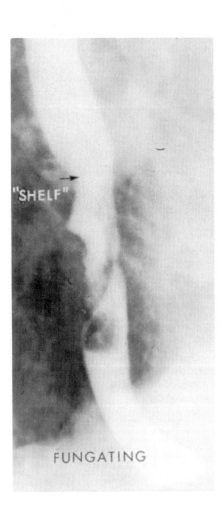

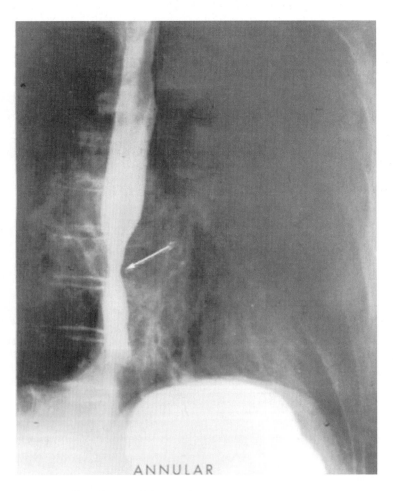

**FIGURE 3-30.** Esophagogram demonstrating squamous cell carcinoma of the esophagus.

*IMAGING*

- The only useful information on plain x-ray is presence of free intraperitoneal air in cases of penetrating visceral injuries.
- Ultrasound is useful for rapid screening (focused assessment with sonography for trauma [FAST] scan) (Figs. 3-31 and 3-32).
- CT is the imaging modality of choice (Fig. 3-33–3-35).

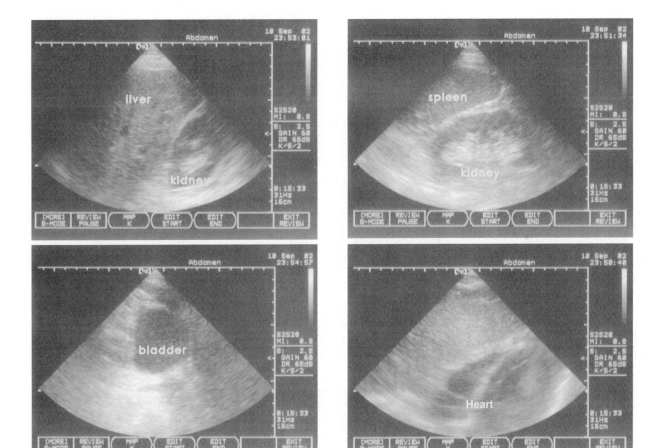

**FIGURE 3-31.** Ultrasound demonstrating normal FAST exam.

(Reproduced, with permission, from Stead LG, Stead SM, Kaufman MS: *First Aid for the Surgery Clerkship.* New York: McGraw-Hill, 2004: 100.)

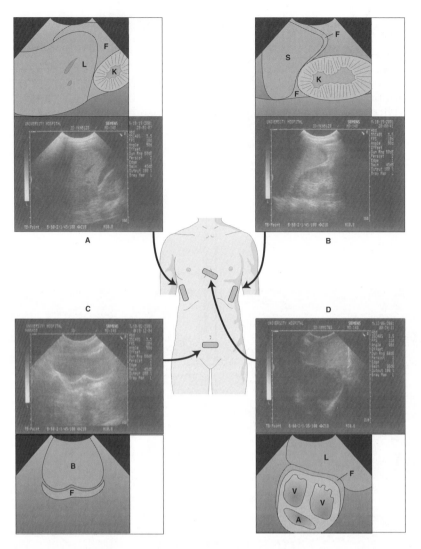

**FIGURE 3-32. Illustration of the four views for the FAST exam and where fluid would be seen in each view.**

A, atrium; B, bladder; F, fluid; K, kidney; L, liver; S, spleen; V, ventricle. (Reproduced, with permission, from Stone CK, Humphries RL. *Current Diagnosis & Treatment: Emergency Medicine, 6th ed.* New York: McGraw-Hill, 2008.)

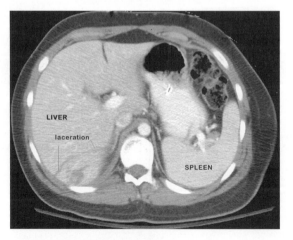

**FIGURE 3-33. CT demonstrating liver laceration.**

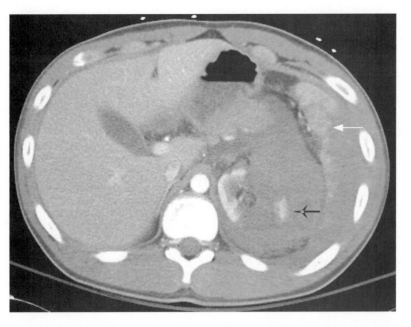

**FIGURE 3-34. Axial CT of the abdomen revealing extensive left renal hematoma and laceration (solid white arrow).**

Also note the splenic laceration with subcapsular hematoma (open black arrow).

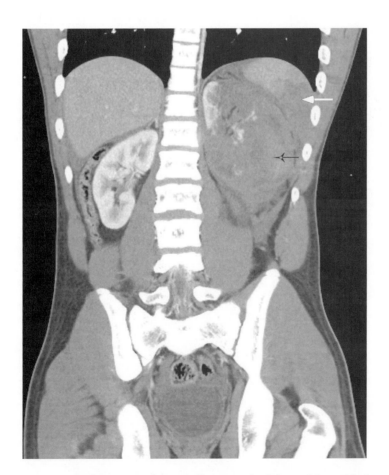

**FIGURE 3-35. Coronal reconstruction revealing extensive left renal (open black arrow) and splenic injuries (solid white arrow).**

# Genitourinary Radiology

**Abdominal X-ray (Kidney/Ureter/Bladder [KUB])**

See Figure 4-1.
- It may be the first diagnostic test to assess the genitourinary system.
- Rule out pregnancy in females of reproductive age group.

See Chapter 3 (Gastrointestinal Radiology) for how to read a plain film (KUB).

### INDICATIONS FOR KUB IN EVALUATION OF THE GU SYSTEM

- Kidney stones (Fig. 4-1).
- Free air indicating perforated viscera. Free air may be visualized under the domes of the diaphragm in an upright view (Fig. 3-13). In sick patients, lateral decubitus view is helpful.
- Abnormal calcifications (Fig. 4-2).
- Renal agenesis (see normal renal outlines in Figure 4-2).
- **Ascites:** Look for obliteration of peritoneal fat pads, displacement of bowel loops (Fig. 4-3).
- **Bowel obstruction:** Look for air-fluid levels, dilated bowel loops, obvious points of transition. Small vs. large bowel obstruction (Fig. 3-12).
- Foreign bodies (Fig. 4-4).
- Skeletal pathologies.

### ADVANTAGES

- Quick
- Inexpensive
- Noninvasive
- Easy availability

### LIMITATIONS

- Renal outline may be obscured by bowel gas.
- Radiation exposure
- No functional information
- Retained barium from other procedures may interfere with visualization.

**Abdominal (Ultrasound [US])**

### ADVANTAGES

- Inexpensive
- Noninvasive. Often used as first-line modality to image the kidneys in cases of acute renal failure.
- It involves no contrast or radiation exposure and is safe in patients with deranged kidney function.

### LIMITATIONS

US provides no functional information

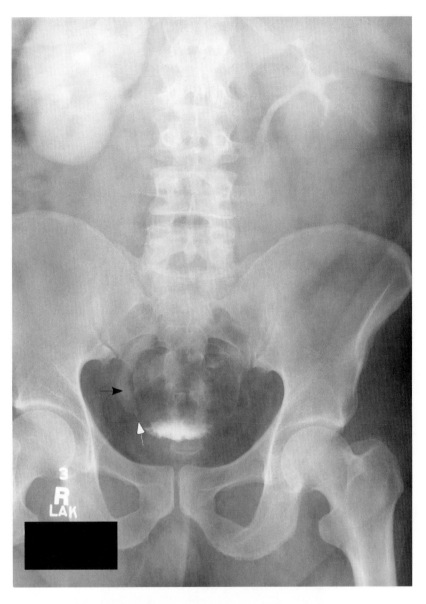

FIGURE 4-1. KUB with contrast, (i.e., intravenous pyelogram, or IVP) demonstrating stone at the uretero-vesicular junction (UVJ) (white arrow). Note dilated ureter proximal to the stone (black arrow).

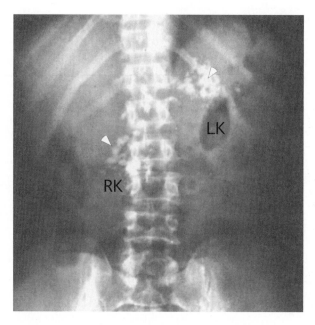

**FIGURE 4-2. KUB demonstrating bilateral adrenal calcifications (black arrows). Can be seen in infections.**

Note normal locations of right kidney (RK) which is lower than the left kidney (LK). (Reproduced, with permission, from Chen MYM, Pope Jr., TL, Ott DJ: *Basic Radiology*. http://accessmedicine.com, McGraw-Hill, 2008.)

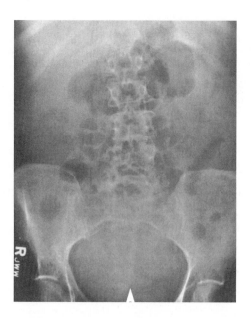

**FIGURE 4-3. KUB demonstrating an increased density in the pelvic cavity with central and upward displacement of bowel loops, and obliteration of peritoneal fat pads due to ascites.**

(Reproduced, with permission, from Chen MYM, Pope Jr., TL, Ott DJ: *Basic Radiology*. http://accessmedicine.com, McGraw-Hill, 2008.)

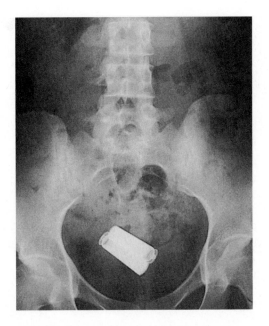

**FIGURE 4-4. KUB demonstrating battery pack in rectum.**

(Reproduced, with permission, from Knoop, Stack & Storrow, 2nd ed. *Atlas of Emergency Medicine*. http://accessmedicine.com, McGraw-Hill, 2008.)

### WHAT TO LOOK FOR IN A RENAL ULTRASOUND (FIG. 4-5)

1. **Kidney size:** Large variation in size based on age. Length ranges from 10-14 cm and breadth 3-5 cm.
2. **Location:** Normal location is retroperitoneal, paraspinal, behind the liver on the right and spleen on the left. Right kidney is lower than the left due to the liver.
3. **Renal outline:** Should normally be smooth. Irregular outline may be from masses or scars.
4. **Corticomedullary differentiation:** Cortex appears hypoechoic (bright) relative to the medulla, which is hypoechoic. In a normal kidney, this differentiation is well maintained, as seen in Figure 4-5.

### INDICATIONS

- **Hydronephrosis:** Appears as calyceal splitting. In cases with distal obstruction, proximal end of dilated ureter may be seen.
- **Calculi:** Appear as echogenic (bright) structures with distal acoustic shadowing.
- **Cysts:** US is extremely useful for delineating cystic vs. solid lesions and defining cyst characteristics (Fig. 4-6).
- Renal masses (Fig. 4-7, angiomyolipoma).
- US guidance may be used for kidney biopsy, e.g., in medical renal disease (Figs. 4-8 and 4-9).
- **Renal artery stenosis:** Combined with Doppler, US is the screening modality of choice for renal artery stenosis (Fig. 4-10).
- Enlarged/ shrunken kidneys: Enlarged kidneys may be seen in Amyloidosis, Multiple myeloma, Diabetes mellitus. Atrophic kidneys may be post obstructive or post infective (Fig. 4-11).

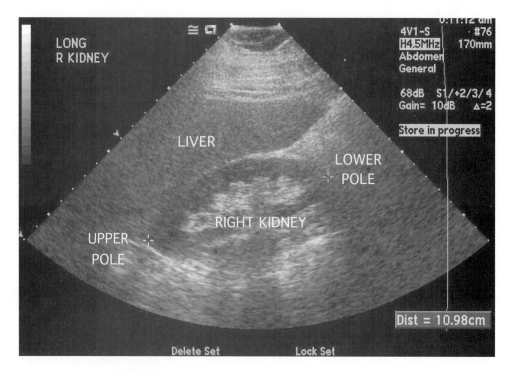

FIGURE 4-5. Ultrasound demonstrating normal kidney.

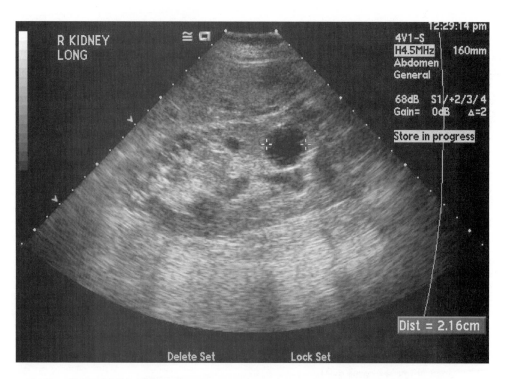

FIGURE 4-6. Ultrasound of the abdomen revealing multiple cysts in the right kidney in a patient with polycystic kidney disease.

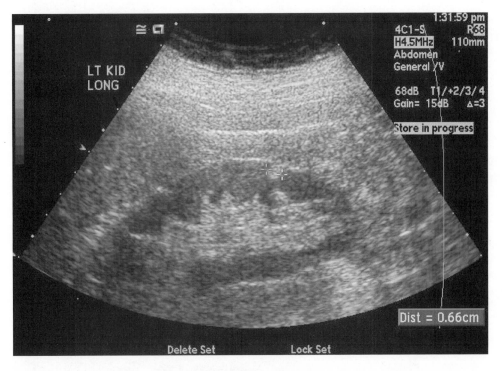

**FIGURE 4-7.** Ultrasound of the abdomen demonstrating an echogenic mass within the left renal cortex (hatchmarks), consistent with an angiomyolipoma.

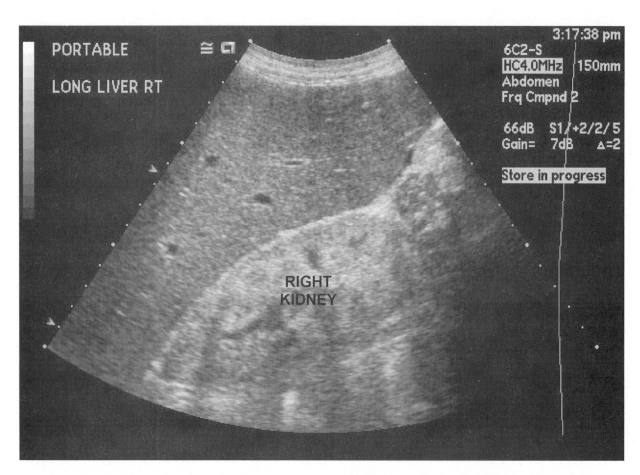

**FIGURE 4-8.** Ultrasound of the abdomen depicting echogenic right kidney in a patient with medical renal disease.

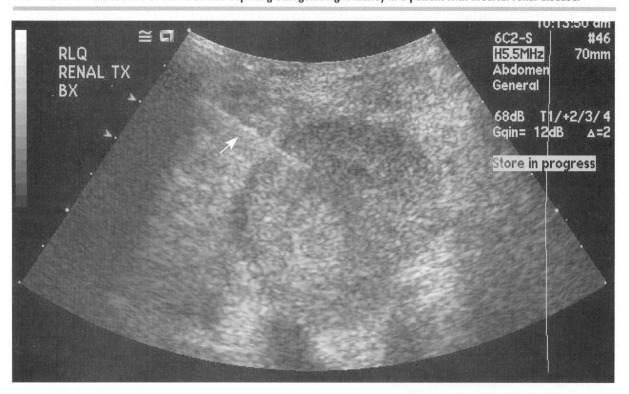

**FIGURE 4-9.** Ultrasound of the abdomen demonstrating biopsy needle (arrow) within lower pole of right kidney.

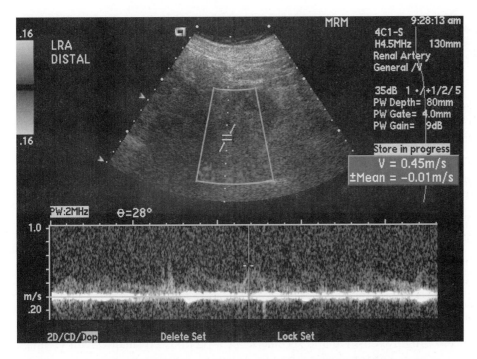

FIGURE 4-10. Ultrasound doppler of the left renal artery depicting diminished distal wave forms in a patient with significant left renal artery stenosis (also see Fig. 4-27, angiogram of bilateral renal artery stenosis).

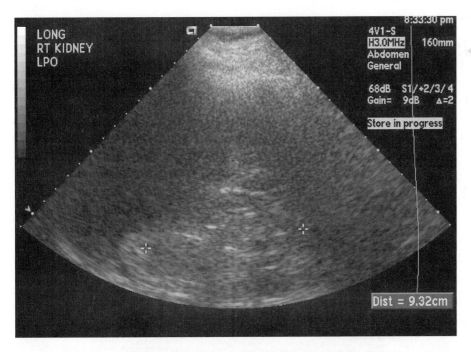

FIGURE 4-11. Ultrasound of the abdomen depicting atrophied right kidney (hatchmarks).

### Abdominal Computed Tomography (CT)

(See Figure 3-3 for normal abdomen/pelvis CT cross section.)

#### ADVANTAGES

- Excellent cross-sectional imaging modality that provides functional information as well.
- It may be done with or without contrast.
- Check kidney function before contrast administration.
- Nonionic contrast preferred because of reduced side effects.

#### LIMITATIONS

- Radiation exposure
- Expensive
- Contrast exposure

#### WHEN TO ORDER ABDOMINAL CT

Three common indications are:
1. **Renal stone disease (painful hematuria):** Noncontrast CT is becoming the gold standard for detection of renal calculi (Fig. 4-12). It is highly sensitive and specific in picking up even small calculi (2 mm). Remember to look for proximal signs of obstruction.
2. **Renal/bladder masses (painless hematuria):** CT can delineate exact extent, characteristics, vascular involvement, lymph node, presence or absence of calcification. *Note:* For bladder masses, cystoscopy may be used for direct visualization of the mass and obtaining biopsy or cauterization of active bleeding sites.
3. **Trauma:** CT is helpful in estimating the degree of trauma. It also provides functional information and is helpful in staging, which is used for prognosis (see Figs. 4-28 and 4-29).

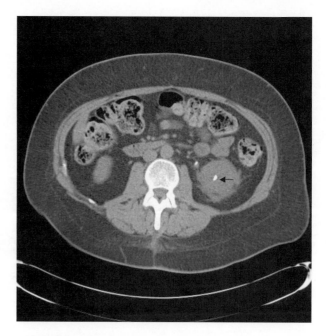

**FIGURE 4-12.** Renal stone (arrow) on noncontrast CT.

## Abdominal MRI

### ADVANTAGES OVER *CT*

- Excellent soft tissue detail (Fig. 4-13).
- Better for staging genitourinary malignancies.
- No radiation exposure.
- Provides functional information in patients with contraindications to iodinated contrast.

### LIMITATIONS

- Expensive
- Limited availability

MRI is extremely useful for diagnosing intrauterine genitourinary anomalies like renal agenesis, polycystic kidneys, which may be missed on antenatal US.

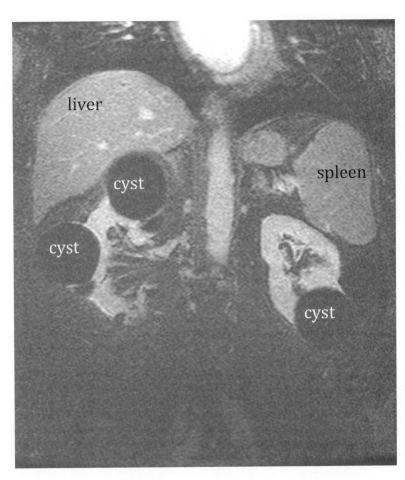

FIGURE 4-13. **MRI of the abdomen in a patient allergic to iodine depicting multiple cysts in bilateral kidneys.**

### CONTRAST STUDIES

Contrast agents used are iodinated and may be intravenous (IV) or intracavitary (IC).

- Excretory urogram, retrograde urethrography, retrograde pyelography, and voiding cystourethrogram (VCUG) (Fig. 4-15).
- Excretory urogram is the most widely used. Special modifications include Furosemide challenge to rule out pelviureteric junction (PUJ) obstruction.

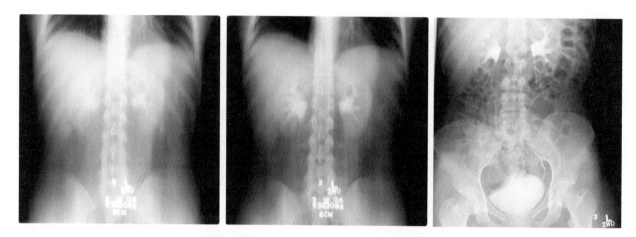

**FIGURE 4-14.** Excretory urethrogram (also known as an intravenous pyelogram, or IVP).

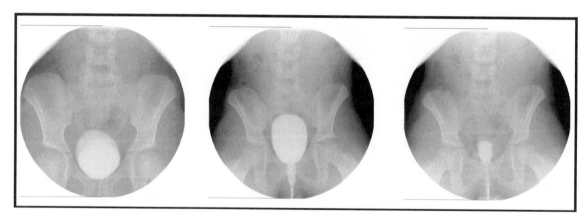

**FIGURE 4-15.** Normal voiding cystourethrogram (VCUG).

- Renal scans are particularly helpful to evaluate renal function in patients with contrast allergy/sensitivity.
- Types of nuclear scans include DMSA, Tc-MAG 3 (Fig. 4-16).
    - DMSA scans are indicated for localizing renal tissue, for example, in cases with ectopic kidneys.
    - Tc-MAG 3 are used in the following cases:
        - Obstructive uropathy (Fig. 4-17).
        - Renovascular hypertension.
        - Renal transplant evaluation.

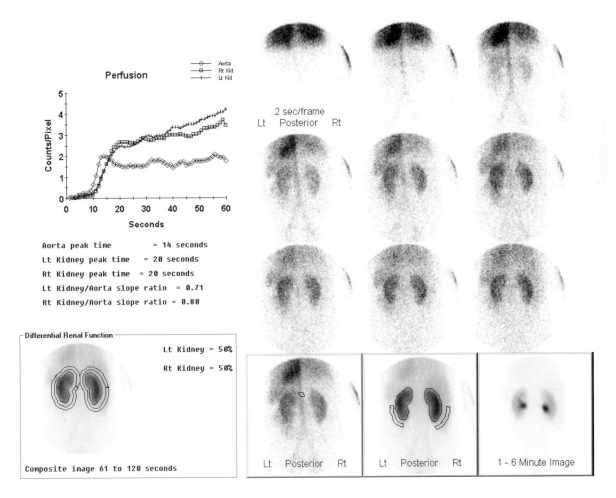

**FIGURE 4-16. MAG 3 (Mercapto Acetyl Tri Glycine) renal scan.**

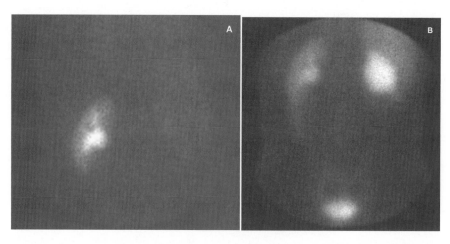

**FIGURE 4-17. Tc-MAG 3 kidney scan (A: Pre-furosemide, and B: Post-furosemide). A shows minimal cortical activity. B shows retention of tracer within a dilated collecting system in a patient with right obstructive uropathy.**

▶ **RENAL CALCULUS DISEASE**

*CAUSES*

Metabolic, structural defects, and recurrent infections

*IMAGING FINDINGS*

Noncontrast CT of the abdomen is emerging as the imaging test of choice.

Remember: Ureteric calculi within the pelvis need to be distinguished from phleboliths. "Rim sign" is soft tissue density around the hyperdense lesion and represents ureteric wall edema.

- Contrast enhancement may be used for functional assessment. X-ray KUB may still be the standard initial study. Only radiopaque stones can be detected with x-ray. Excretory urogram can demonstrate the level of obstruction. Persistent nephrogram and contrast column are highly suggestive of obstruction.
- Rule out associated conditions and causes of medullary calcification:
  - Renal tubular acidosis.
  - Hyperparathyroidism.
  - Sarcoidosis.
  - Hyperoxaluria.
  - Hypercalciuria.
  - **Infectious causes:** Tuberculosis, xanthogranulomatous pyelonephritis (usually associated with *Proteus* infections, needs to be differentiated from malignancy).
  - Rarely, calcifications may be seen with malignancies, especially neuroblastoma, Wilms' tumor.

Interventions for obstructive calculi:

- **Percutaneous lithotripsy:** The breaking of a calculus by shock waves or crushing with a surgical instrument in the urinary system into pieces small enough to be voided or washed out—called also *litholapaxy, lithotrity*
- **Percutaneous nephrostomy:** Placement of a stent from the renal pelvis to the outside of the body
- **Percutaneous nephrolithotomy:** Surgical removal of the stone.
- Retrograde stone extraction for bladder or lower ureteric calculi.

*CAUSES*

Clinical history is the most important part of the workup.

*IMAGING FINDINGS*

- Ultrasound is the first-line imaging test. Rule out obstruction and reversible causes and vascular pathology like renal artery stenosis.
- Noncontrast CT may be needed for detecting ureteric calculi. Contrast enhancement gives functional assessment.
- Nuclear studies are helpful in the assessment of post-transplant patients.

► URINARY TRACT INFECTIONS

*CAUSES*

- **Most common pathogens:** Gram-negative rods, disseminated fungal infections in immunocompromised/AIDS hosts.
- Renal tuberculosis is rare within the United States (Fig. 4-18).
- **Rare infections:** Disseminated fungal, tuberculosis, schistosomiasis, and xanthogranulomatous pyelonephritis.
- **Spectrum:** Uncomplicated UTI → Cystitis → Pyelonephritis → Perinephric abscess → Pyelonephrosis.
- May be complicated or uncomplicated.
- Lower tract infections are usually uncomplicated.
- Routine imaging not indicated in uncomplicated UTIs.
- Most common pathogens: Gram-negative rods; disseminated fungal infections in immunocompromised/AIDS hosts.
- Renal tuberculosis is rare within the United States ( Fig. 4-18).
- Rare infections: Disseminated fungal, tuberculosis, schistosomiasis, and xanthogranulomatous pyelonephritis.
- Indications for imaging: Recurrent infections, complicated course, deranged kidney function, nonresponsive to susceptible antimicrobial treatment.

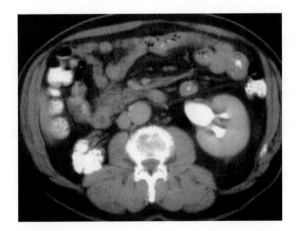

**FIGURE 4-18. Abdominal CT showing densely calcified nonfunctioning right kidney (putty kidney) due to longstanding tuberculosis.**

1. **Acute pyelonephritis (Fig. 4-19)**
   - Limited role of imaging in diagnosis and management of these patients.
   - Ultrasound
     - Can rule out structural defects and abscess formation in recurrent and nonresponding cases. Kidneys may have a globally hypoechoic (darker) appearance on ultrasound in acute cases.
   - On dimercaptosuccinic acid (DMSA)
     - Peripheral defects can denote edema or scarring.
   - Computed tomography (CT)
     - Peripheral wedge-shaped hypodense areas, which need to be differentiated from infarcts.
     - Diabetics are predisposed to development of emphysematous pyelonephritis and cystitis (Fig. 4-20), which is a surgical emergency and needs timely debridement. Plain x-rays can diagnose air within the renal region. However, it may be difficult to delineate from bowel gas. CT is confirmatory and assesses exact extent of involvement.

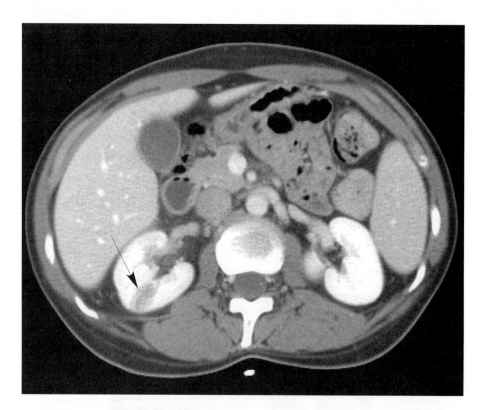

**FIGURE 4-19.** CT abdomen demonstrating nonenchancing focal areas in right kidney compatible with pyelonephritis.

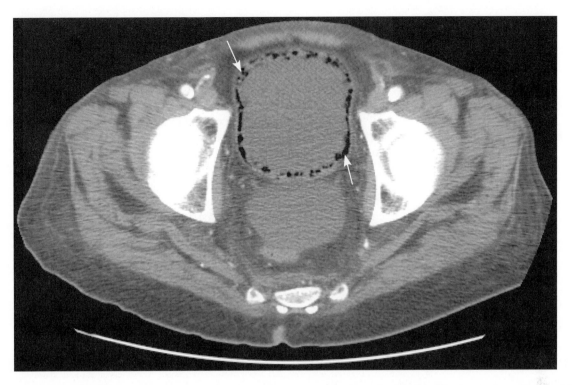

**FIGURE 4-20.** CT abdomen demonstrating air in the lumen and within the wall of the bladder (arrows) consistent with emphysematous cystitis.

### 2. Perinephric abscess (Fig. 4-21)

- Rare complication. Abscess formation around the kidney.
- Pyelonephrosis implies abscess formation within renal parenchyma.

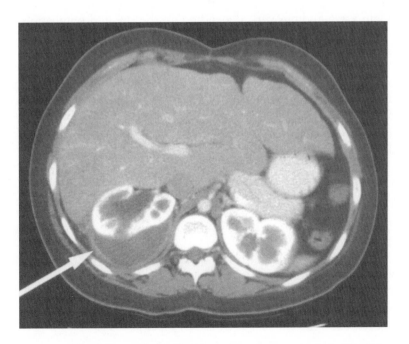

**FIGURE 4-21.** CT demonstrating peripherally enhancing abscess around the kidney (arrow).

(Reproduced, with permission, from Tanagho EA, McAnnich JW: *Smith's General Urology*, 6th ed. http://accessmedicine.com, McGraw-Hill, 2008.)

3. **Renal tuberculosis**
   - Tuberculosis of the urinary tract is an important clinical problem because of its nonspecific clinical presentations and varying imaging appearances.
   - Kidneys are generally involved secondary to the hematogenous spread of the *Mycobacterium* from a primary pulmonary focus.
   - Tubercle bacilli form renal cortical granulomas, which coalesce to form cavities. Cavities may rupture and communicate with the pelvicalyceal system.
   - The end result of the disease is destruction, loss of function, and calcification of the entire kidney.
   - In later stages, common findings include a deformed renal outline, calcifications, cavitations, and stricture formation.
   - Ultrasound may be helpful in demonstrating calyceal dilation and obstruction.
   - CT will demonstrate focal caliectasis, hydronephrosis, calcifications, cortical thinning, and soft tissue masses.
   - In early disease, excretory urography is the imaging modality of choice as it may detect changes within a single calyx.

> ▶ **RENAL MASSES**

## Benign Renal Masses

### ANGIOMYOLIPOMAS

#### *CAUSES*

They may occur sporadically or as part of syndromes

#### *IMAGING FINDINGS*

- Plain x-ray findings vary, depending on the size and number. These include defect in renal contour, lucency due to underlying fat, and occasionally calcification.
- On ultrasound, angiomyolipomas appear most commonly echogenic due to tissue interfaces and fat. There may occasionally be evidence of cavitation and calcification (Fig. 4-22).
- CT scan is helpful in demonstrating Hounsfield Unit (HU) value compatible with fat. Potential complications include hematuria and retroperitoneal hemorrhage.

### ONCOCYTOMA

#### *IMAGING FINDINGS*

- Characteristic radiologic feature is central stellate scar composed of fibrous tissue.
- Angiography reveals a distinct "spoke wheel pattern" constituted by homogenous blush and enhancing blood vessels.

- Most common benign renal masses.
- As the name suggests, these are composed of varying proportions of fat, vascular, and smooth muscles.

- Is a rare type of renal adenoma.
- Usual age of presentation is 60–70 years.

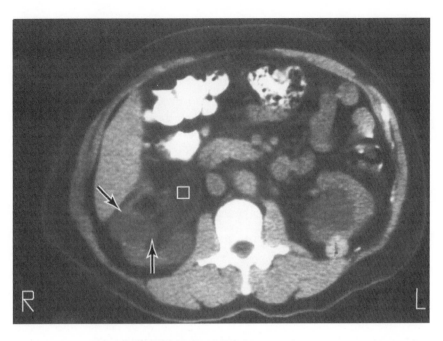

**FIGURE 4-22. CT demonstrating angiomyolipoma.**

(Reproduced, with permission, from Tanagho EA, McAnnich JW: *Smith's General Urology*, 6th ed. http://accessmedicine.com, McGraw-Hill, 2008.)

## Malignant Renal Masses

### 1. RENAL CELL CARCINOMA (RCC)

#### *IMAGING FINDINGS*

- Excretory urogram may reveal mass effect in renal regions with calyceal splaying hydronephrosis. In smaller masses, however, it may be entirely normal.
- Ultrasound is excellent in differentiating cystic from solid lesions; however, it is inferior in detecting tumor extent and staging. Smaller solid isoechoic lesions may be entirely missed.
- CT scan is the imaging modality of choice for the staging of renal cell carcinoma. CT features vary according to the size and type of lesion. Most commonly, these appear as heterodense, heterogenously enhancing intrarenal masses, which may cause irregularity in renal contour. Other features include calyceal splaying, stretching, distortion of intrarenal architecture, obstruction, vascular invasion, and lymph nodal and distant metastases (Fig. 4-23).
- MRI is superior to CT for imaging the staging of more advanced disease. It is more advantageous in detecting exact extent of tumor thrombi and has replaced venography for detecting venous involvement.
- Imaging plays an extremely crucial role in preoperative planning and prognosis.

- The most common renal malignancy.
- Recent advances in cross-sectional imaging have enabled early detection of disease in localized stage.

A solid renal mass is presumed malignant (RCC) unless proven otherwise. Triad of RCC (pain, flank mass, hematuria) is seen in 10% of patients.

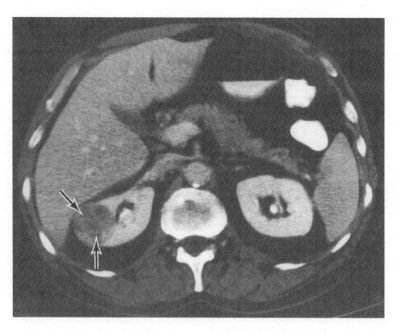

**FIGURE 4-23. Contrast CT of abdomen and pelvis demonstrating RCC.**

(Reproduced, with permission, from Tanagho EA, McAninch JW: *Smith's General Urology*, 6th ed. http://accessmedicine.com, McGraw-Hill, 2008.)

- Arises from the urothelial lining.
- Is often synchronous and metachronous
- Most common kind of bladder cancer. Grossly appears as polypoid peduculated or sessile mass within the urinary bladder.

## 2. TRANSITIONAL CELL CARCINOMA

### LOCATION

May arise anywhere from the collecting system to the urinary bladder.

### IMAGING FINDINGS

- Excretory urogram is most sensitive in diagnosing early lesions involving the collecting systems. When large, they mimic RCC. CT is helpful in delineating extent.
- For accurate staging, cross-sectional imaging with CT/MRI is employed. MRI is more useful than CT in estimating tumor invasion and perivesical fat involvement. Also, MRI is more useful in delineating tumor mass from scar tissue in postoperative cases.
- Cystoscopy remains an extremely useful imaging technique for bladder cancer, which allows interventions for diagnostic or therapeutic purposes.

## ADRENAL ADENOMA

- Is a common benign tumor of the adrenal cortex. Occasionally it is functional, and causes an endocrinopathy.
- The typical imaging features of an adrenal adenoma are those of a small homogeneous mass.
- They are often not detected at ultrasound. At CT, which should be the first imaging study, the adrenal adenomas have a smooth rounded appearance with a low density (Fig. 4.24). An attenuation value of under 30 HU on a post contrast (1 hour) has a high sensitivity and specificity for the diagnosis of adenoma.
- On MRI, adenomas are usually isointense or hypointense to liver on both T1- and T2-weighted images. The tumors enhance after intravenous gadolinium.

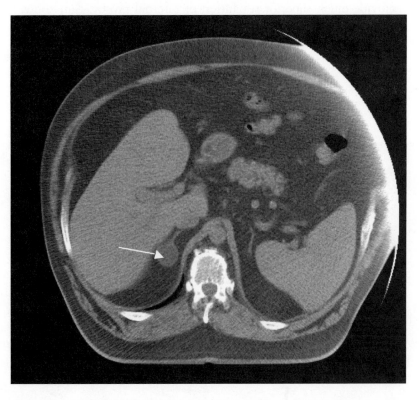

**FIGURE 4-24. Abdominal CT showing right kidney adrenal adenoma (arrow).**

### Benign Prostatic Hypertrophy (BPH)

- BPH has a high prevalence that increases with age.
- BPH arises in the central gland while prostate cancer typically arises in the peripheral gland.
- Ultrasound is a noninvasive, cost-efficient imaging modality and is often the first line imaging study. It may be used for biopsy guidance for definitive diagnosis. Approaches used may be transrectal or transabdominal.
- Sonographic appearance of BPH is variable. BPH may appear as a single or as multiple nodules within the transition zone which may be surrounded by a thin hypoechoic rim that clearly delineates them from the adjoining tissue (Fig. 4-25). The nodules may be hypo, iso- or hyperechoic with respect to the surrounding gland. Unlike prostate cancer, they do not cause capsular disruption. US may also be used to image the kidneys in order to rule out back pressure changes.
- MRI is not routinely used for imaging as is very costly. It does however provide much superior resolution of internal prostatic anatomy, better delineation of glandular from stromal tissue in the prostate, and an accurate estimate of prostate volume.
- CT has extremely limited application due to its inability to define intraprostatic zonal anatomy.

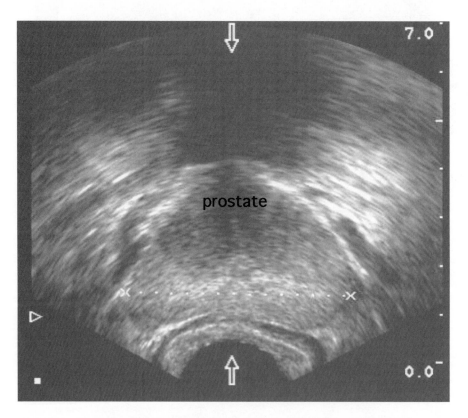

**FIGURE 4-25. Endorectal US showing benign hypertrophy of the prostate gland.**

## Testicular Torsion

- Torsion is twisting of the testis within the scrotum causing venous obstruction and eventually arterial obstruction and vascular compromise.
- It is most commonly seen around the time of puberty but also occurs in neonates. Intrauterine torsion has also been described.
- Ultrasound scanning is quick, readily available and the imaging modality of choice in these patients. It shows a swollen and hypoechoic testis in the early phase with a sympathetic hydroele (Fig. 4-26). With increasing duration, secondary hemorrhage may cause areas of increased echogenicity.
- Doppler ultrasound of the cord shows reduced arterial signal. Absent flow within the testis strongly suggests torsion.
- Technetium pertechnetate scanning has been used to demonstrate hypoperfusion of the testis but is now replaced by ultrasound.

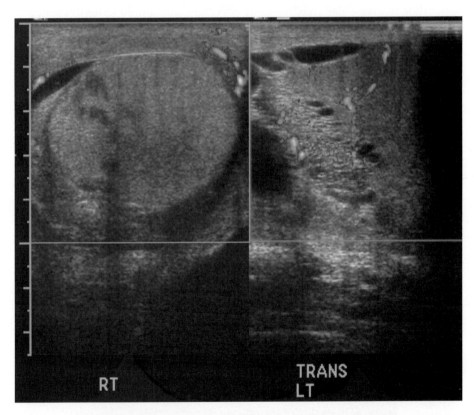

**FIGURE 4-26.** Doppler ultrasound of bilateral testes shows swollen up right testis with hypoechoic areas within and absence of flow suggesting testicular torsion with necrosis.

### Renal Artery Stenosis

- Atherosclerosis and fibrosing lesions of the walls of the vessels (fibromuscular dysplasia) are the most common causes of RAS; atherosclerosis being the most frequent cause.

- Features on hypertensive urography, which is no longer performed include disparity in the size of the two kidneys with delayed appearance of the contrast medium into the calyces. Also, urine flow is decreased resulting in a spidery pyelogram. The affected side may show greater or lesser radiodensity than the other side. Ureteric notching due to collaterals may be seen.

- Doppler ultrasound is used to study renal artery velocities and waveforms. Increased renal: aortic velocity ratio (≥ 3.5), peak renal artery velocity of ≥ 100 cm/sec, slow rise to peak velocity (pulsus tardus) are some of the features which may be noted.

- Nuclear imaging using Tc-MAG 3 before and after the administration of captopril (an angiotensin-converting enzyme (ACE) inhibitor) may be used. A positive ACE inhibition scintigraphy examination indicates that renovascular hypertension is present and implies the existence of hemodynamically significant renal artery stenosis.

- Angiography is used for confirmation of diagnosis. Findings include a delayed nephrogram and a stenosed segment with poststenotic dilatation (Fig. 4-27). Renal vein sampling can detect the increased renin levels, which localize to the involved side in the setting of renovascular hypertension.

- Today, CT angiography with MIP and MR angiography with (3D) dynamic gadolinium enhanced and phase contrast techniques have emerged as noninvasive methods for the evaluation of vascular stenosis.

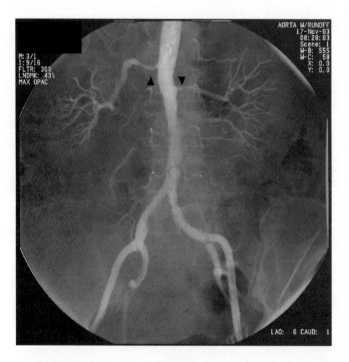

**FIGURE 4-27.** Angiogram demonstrating bilateral renal artery stenoses at the origin (arrows). Accessory renal artery is noted on the left side.

# Obstetrics and Gynecology

- Radiosensitivity in pregnancy varies according to gestational period and amount of radiation exposure.
- Potential hazards of ionizing radiation:
  - Congenital malformations
  - Prenatal death
  - Growth restriction
  - Neurological defects
  - Increased cancer risk
  - First 2 weeks: Doses > 5 rads cause damage (usually miscarriage).
  - 3 to 15 weeks: Most sensitive stage is between 8 and 15 weeks. Threshold dose is 30 rads before any apparent effect. Effects at this stage are primarily neurological, like mental retardation.
  - 16 to 26 weeks: Adverse effects seen only with extremely large doses of radiation exposure.
  - Beyond 26 weeks: Radiosensitivity similar to that of newborn. Main adverse effect is small increase in likelihood of cancer in later life.

## Ultrasound in Pregnancy

- Ultrasound scanning is an integral part of antenatal care and is considered to be a safe, accurate, noninvasive, and cost-effective investigation in pregnancy and fetal assessment (Fig. 5-2).
- Approaches may be transabdominal or transvaginal.
- Full bladder required for acoustic window and good visualization of pelvic contents in transabdominal approach.
- Its main uses in early pregnancy are for:
  - Diagnosis of early pregnancy
  - Confirmation of site of pregnancy (intrauterine vs. ectopic).
  - Assessment of vaginal bleeding and viability of the fetus
  - Evaluation of fetal number
  - The gestational sac can be visualized as early as 4½ weeks of gestation. Its location is usually fundal and has a regular outline with thick echogenic walls (Fig. 5-1).
  - The yolk sac is seen within the echolucent gestational sac at about 5 weeks.
  - The fetal pole can be observed and measured by about 5½ weeks. Fetal heartbeat is usually seen and detected by pulsed Doppler ultrasound at about 6 weeks.
  - Crown-to-rump length (CRL) measurement can be made between 7 and 13 weeks and gives a very accurate estimation of the gestational age. In early cases if the fetal node is seen, mean sac diameter (MSD) is used for pregnancy dating purpose. From the second trimester onwards, biparietal diameter (BPD), head circumference (HC), abdominal circumference (AC), and femur length (FL) are the parameters most commonly used for maturity assessment (Fig. 5-3).
  - Visualization of the adnexal regions may show corpus luteal cysts.
  - Observation of internal os and cervical length measurement may be of value in assessment of cervical incompetence.
  - More fetal structures such as the face become apparent on third trimester ultrasound (Fig. 5-4).

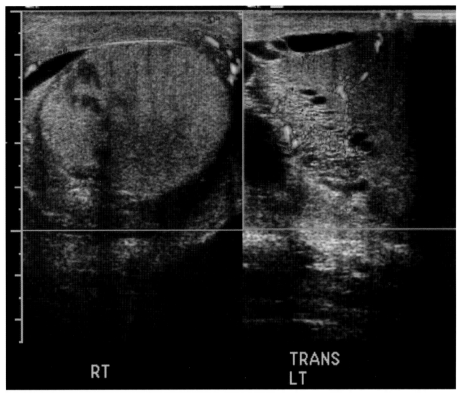

**FIGURE 4-26.** Doppler ultrasound of bilateral testes shows swollen up right testis with hypoechoic areas within and absence of flow suggesting testicular torsion with necrosis.

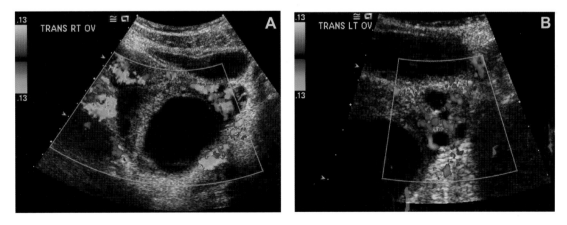

**FIGURE 5-11. Sonogram of ovaries.**

Panel (A) is an ultrasound Doppler depicting hypoechoic enlarged right ovary with a large cystic area and lack of vascular signal on Doppler, consistent with torsion. Panel (B) shows normal left side ovary with normal vasculature.

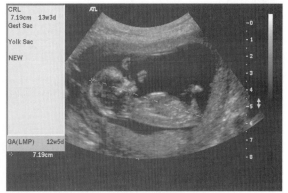
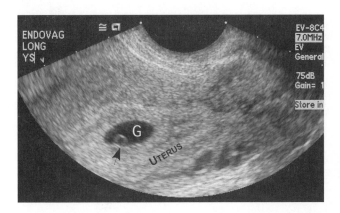

**FIGURE 5-1. First-trimester ultrasound.**

Panel on left is an endovaginal scan depicting the intrauterine gestational sac (G), the yolk sac (arrow), and the uterus (outlined). Panel on the right is a transabdominal scan depicting the crown-to-rump length (dashed line).

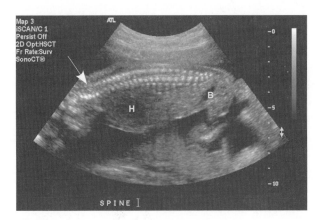
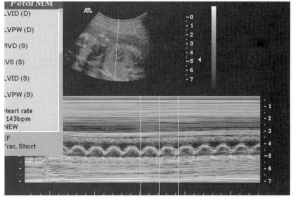

**FIGURE 5-2. Second-trimester ultrasound.**

Left panel: Transabdominal ultrasound depicting longitudinal view of fetus in the second trimester. Note bladder (B), heart (H), diaphragm (outlined) and craniovertebral junction (arrow). Right panel: M-mode ultrasound depicting normal cardiac activity.

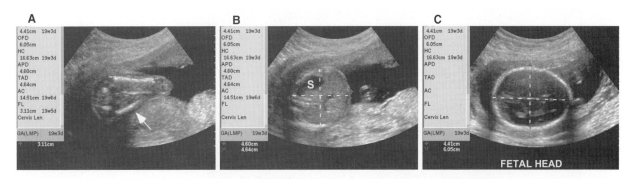

**FIGURE 5-3. Second-trimester ultrasound showing standard fetal measurements for fetal maturity.**

(A) shows measurement of femur length (FL). (B) shows measurement of fetal abdominal circumference (AC). Note stomach(s). (C) shows measurement of head circumference (HC) and biparietal diameter (BPD).

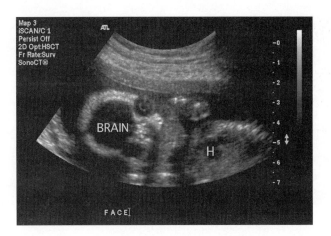

**FIGURE 5-4.** Third-trimester ultrasound depicting normal structures of fetal face.

Note heart (H).

## Ectopic Pregnancy

- Ectopic pregnancy is a potentially life-threatening emergency. It is the second leading cause of maternal mortality, and its incidence in the United States in about 1 in 100 pregnancies.
- This diagnosis should be considered in any pregnant patient who presents within the 1st trimester with abdominal pain or vaginal bleeding.
- Imaging findings (Fig. 5-5):
    - Presence of an echogenic adnexal mass
    - An empty uterus
    - Free fluid in the pelvis
    - Cardiac activity outside the uterus confirms diagnosis
    - Treatment consists of hemodynamic stabilization, $Rh_0(D)$ immunoglobulin for Rh-negative women, and treatment of the ectopic mass either surgically or medically with methotrexate.

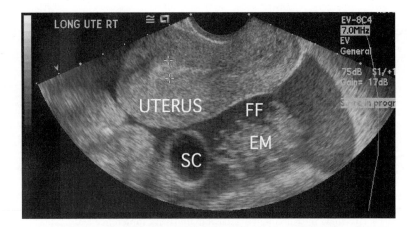

**FIGURE 5-5.** Transvaginal sonogram demonstrating an ectopic pregnancy.

Note the large amount of free fluid (FF) in the pelvis. No intrauterine pregnancy was seen. A large complex echogenic mass (EM) was seen in the left adnexa, consistent with an ectopic pregnancy. A simple cyst (SC) is also seen, in the right adnexa. The area within the uterus represents a small fibroid.

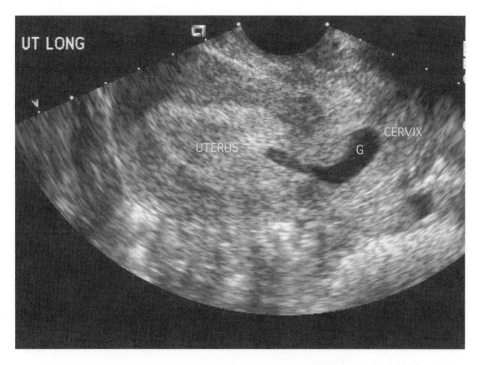

UT LONG

UTERUS      CERVIX

 G

**FIGURE 5-6.** Endovaginal sonogram showing impending spontaneous abortion.

## MRI in Pregnancy

- Generally considered safe in pregnancy
- Should be avoided in first trimester if possible because safety has not been fully established for this period
- Gadolinium (MRI contrast agent) must be strictly avoided because it has been shown to be teratogenic in animal studies.

## CT in Pregnancy (Fig. 5-7)

- CT scanning is, in general, not recommended for pregnant women because of potential risk to the baby.
- However, CT scan may be warranted when necessary for evaluation of the mother in the case of multitrauma, where the risk outweighs the benefit.

Sonographic signs suggesting an abortion/miscarriage are (Fig. 5-6):

- An empty gestational sac with an irregular lining
- A low-lying gestational sac within the lower uterine segment or the uterocervical region
- Absence of cardiac activity beyond 6 weeks of gestation
- Abnormal hyperechoic material within the uterine cavity

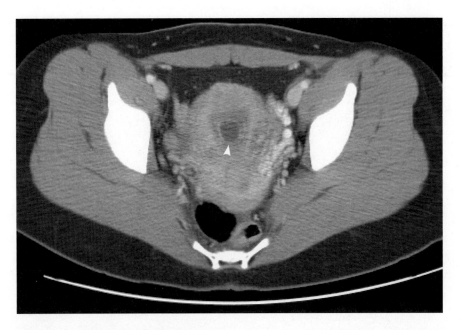

**FIGURE 5-7. CT scan in a pregnant woman.**

Note gestational sac (arrowhead).

## ▶ IMAGING OF THE FEMALE GENITAL TRACT

### Ultrasound

- Most frequently used
- Advantages: No radiation exposure, good visualization, easy accessibility, low cost

### Hysterosalpingogram (Fig. 5-8)

- Contrast study to visualize the uterus and fallopian tubes
- Method: Instillation of contrast via a cannula inserted in the uterus through transvaginal approach
- Normal hysterosalpingogram delineates smooth uterine contour with bilateral tubes and bilateral free intraperitoneal spillage of contrast.
- A blocked tube will result in contrast flowing into peritoneal cavity (Fig. 5-9).
- Precautions: Rule out pregnancy.

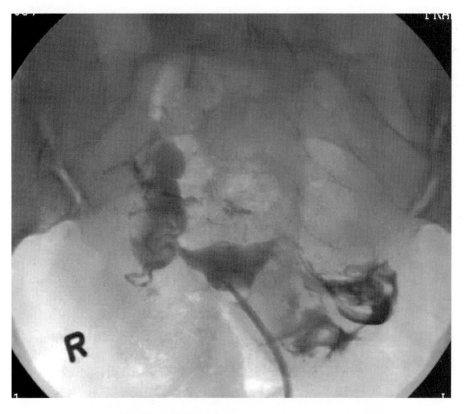

**FIGURE 5-8.** Normal hysterosalpingogram.

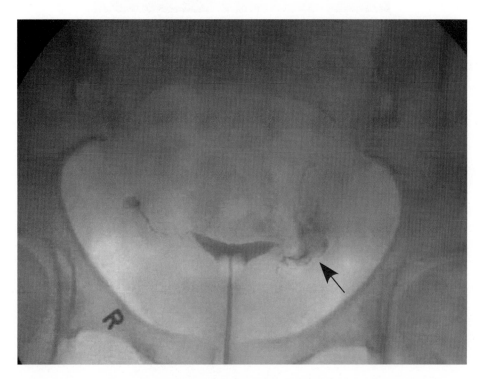

**FIGURE 5-9.** Hysterosalpingogram showing right-sided tubal block with free flow of contrast material into the peritoneal cavity on the left (arrow).

## Cysts

### *FUNCTIONAL*

- Benign
- No treatment or serial imaging needed in asymptomatic cases

### *NEOPLASTIC*

Dermoid cyst of right ovary in an asymptomatic young woman. Note that left ovary appears normal in size with evidence of an ovarian follicle (Fig. 5-10).

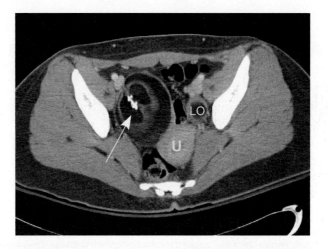

**FIGURE 5-10.** **Pelvic CT demonstrating large dermoid cysts in the right ovary.**

Note the hyperdense (white) tooth. The hypodense areas within the right ovary represent fat. Note also the normal left ovary (LO), and uterus (U).

## Torsion

### CAUSE

Twisting of the ovary around its pedicle

### IMAGING

Ultrasound may reveal affected ovary to be enlarged and hypoechoic. Doppler reveals lack of vascular flow signal (Fig. 5-11).

Ovarian torsion:
- Seen in young females. Rare in premenarchal and postmenopausal women.
- Clinical presentation may be nonspecific. Some may present with acute lower quadrant abdominal pain with nausea and vomiting.
- Treatment is surgical.

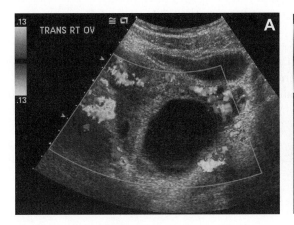
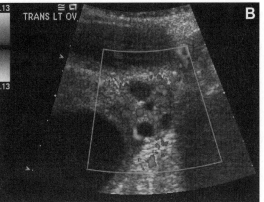

**FIGURE 5-11. Sonogram of ovaries.**

Panel (A) is an ultrasound Doppler depicting hypoechoic enlarged right ovary with a large cystic area and lack of vascular signal on Doppler, consistent with torsion. Panel (B) shows normal left side ovary with normal vasculature.

### Fibroids

Fibroids (leiomyomas) are benign tumors of smooth muscle cell origin and are the most common uterine masses.

#### LOCATION

Fibroids are classified as intramural, submucosal, or subserosal on the basis of their position in relation to the uterine wall.

#### IMAGING

- They may be an incidental finding on pelvic sonograms done for other purposes. On ultrasound, they generally appear as well-demarcated heteroechoic masses. They may show foci of calcification. Ultrasound is a useful and safe imaging modality; however, it is of limited value when the fibroids are small or when the uterus is retroverted. It may not always be possible to differentiate a subserous fibroid from an adnexal pathology on ultrasound. Endovaginal ultrasound better demonstrates their internal architecture as compared to transabdominal scans (Fig. 5-12).
- CT features include focal/multifocal heterodense solid masses. They may be lobulated. Focal calcifications may be seen. Irregular low-density areas within are generally suggestive of necrosis.
- On MRI, leiomyomas are seen as well-circumscribed masses of similar or slightly low T1 signal intensity and homogeneously low T2 signal intensity, relative to the adjacent myometrium. They may be seen to cause distortion of the endometrial cavity. MRI is definitely superior to ultrasound in the evaluation of uterine fibroids. However, it is more expensive.

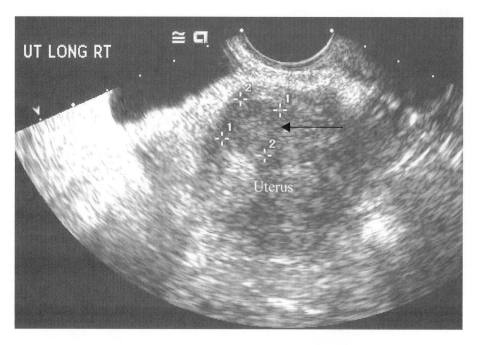

**FIGURE 5-12. Endovaginal sonogram showing uterine fibroid (black arrow).**

## Septate Uterus

### CAUSE

Septate uterus is a congenital anomaly in which a fibrous septum separates the uterine cavity into two compartments.

### IMAGING

- Ultrasound can frequently identify the septum. At hysterosalpingography, a septate uterus is suspected when the two uterine horns are separated by an angle of less than 90 degrees (Fig. 5-13).
- The fibrous nature of the septum is best confirmed by MRI, which shows a septum of low signal intensity on both T1- and T2-weighted sequences. The fundal contour is normal.

Septate vs. bicornuate uterus:

- Septate uterus is associated with increased fetal loss in the second trimester. On the other hand, the bicornuate uterus is thought to have little or no clinical effect on pregnancy.
- Septate uterus can be treated by hysteroscopic division, whereas bicornuate uterus requires open surgical repair.

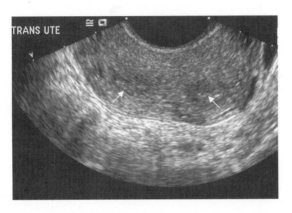

**FIGURE 5-13.** Pelvic ultrasound demonstrating septate uterus (arrows point to the two endometrial stripes).

# Musculoskeletal Radiology

## Plain Films

### WHEN TO ORDER

- Most appropriate screening technique if a fracture is suspected.
- Plain films must be ordered before an MRI, for correct interpretation.

### ADVANTAGES

Can quickly identify if a fracture or other suspected bony pathology is present or not.

### DISADVANTAGES

- A fracture might not be evident on one view and often several different projections are necessary.
- A fracture may be occult. (However, follow-up x-rays in 7–10 days could be obtained if clinical supervision is high.)

## Computed Tomography (CT)

### WHEN TO ORDER

To further evaluate numerous musculoskeletal disorders including neoplasms and subtle or complex fracture.

### ADVANTAGES

- Fast and efficient technique
- Good for bony and articular details
- Both intravenous peripheral contrast and intra-articular contrast may be given.

### DISADVANTAGES

- More radiation than an x-ray
- Metal implants, for example, a hip arthroplasty, cause significant metal artifact.

## Magnetic Resonance Imaging (MRI)

### WHEN TO ORDER

- To evaluate ligament or tendon injury
- To evaluate soft tissue masses
- To evaluate stress fractures and osteomyelitis

### ADVANTAGES

- Excellent for looking at soft tissue, marrow, ligaments, and marrow edema
- Both intra-articular and IV contrast may be used to better delineate anatomy/pathology

### DISADVANTAGES

- Many contraindications including cardiac pacemakers, metallic foreign bodies, cerebral aneurysm clips, electronic devices

- Metallic implants cause artifacts that limit image quality.
- Some patients may be claustrophobic.
- Sedation may be required.

## Fluoroscopy

### WHEN TO ORDER

- Can be used for guidance during biopsy and aspiration
- Used for intra-articular injection of contrast before an MRI or CT if required

### ADVANTAGES

Real-time image guidance

### DISADVANTAGES

Exposure to radiation

## Ultrasound

### WHEN TO ORDER

For further evaluation of joints, soft tissues, and vascular structures

### ADVANTAGES

- Low cost
- Availability

### DISADVANTAGES

Operator dependent

## Dual Energy X-ray Absorptiometry (DEXA)

### WHEN TO ORDER

- Best test to evaluate bone mineral density (BMD)
- Focuses on two main areas consisting of the hip and spine
- Used to assess the strength of bone and probability of fracture in individuals at risk of osteoporosis

### ADVANTAGES

- Preferred technique for measuring BMD
- Easy to perform
- Radiation exposure is low
- Performed in about 10 to 20 minutes

### DISADVANTAGES

- Cost
- Osteoarthritis can confound results of the DEXA scan.

- First determine the location of the fracture. Shafts of long bones are divided into proximal, middle, and distal.
- Check for intra-articular extension of the fracture.
- Look for surrounding soft tissue swelling and/or foreign body.
- Describe fracture type (Fig. 6-1) if appropriate.

*Sample Presentation*

"This is a right wrist x-ray of Mr. Smith. There is a comminuted fracture of the distal radius with intra-articular extension. Associated soft tissue swelling. No additional fractures identified."

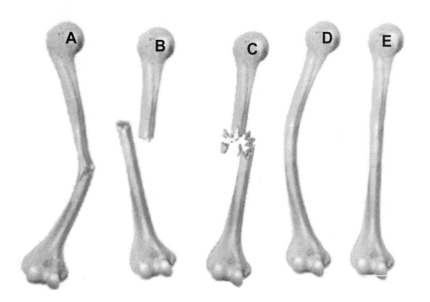

**FIGURE 6-1. Types of fractures.**

A, greenstick fracture; B, displaced fracture; C, comminuted fracture; D, plastic deformity (bowing); E, normal (no fracture).

HIGH-YIELD FACTS

Musculoskeletal Radiology

## Normal Cervical Spine Anatomy (Figs. 6-2—6-6)

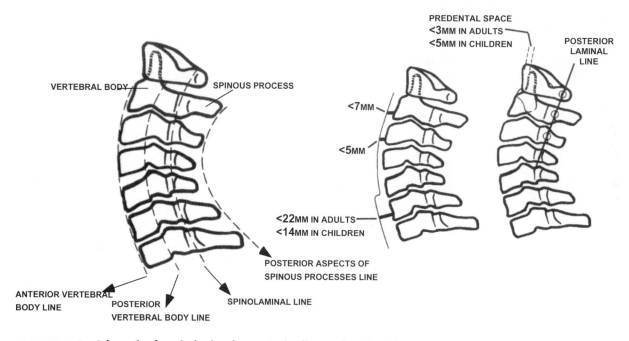

FIGURE 6-2. Schematic of cervical spine demonstrating lines and predental spaces.

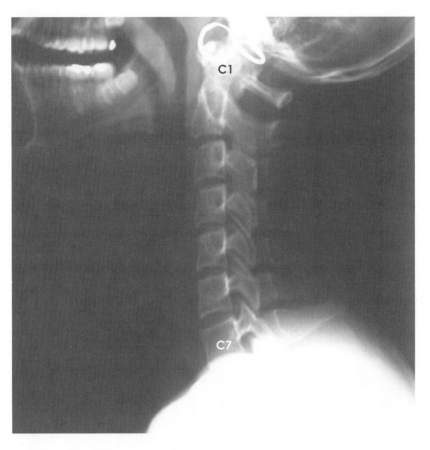

FIGURE 6-3. Normal lateral view of cervical spine.

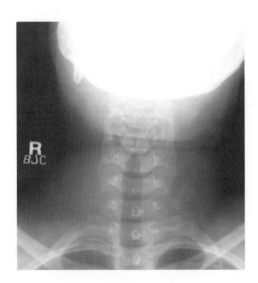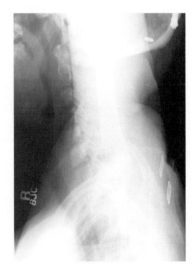

FIGURE 6-4. Normal AP and lateral view of the cervical spine.

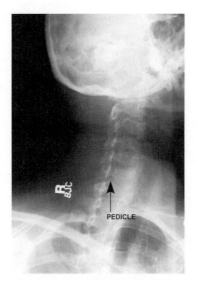
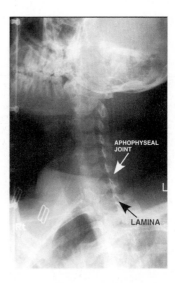

FIGURE 6-5. Normal oblique views of cervical spine.

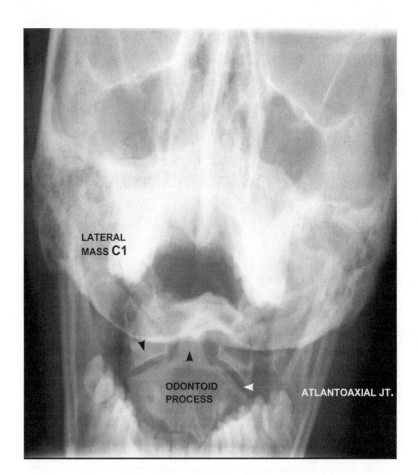

FIGURE 6-6. Normal odontoid views of cervical spine.

## Normal Thoracic Spine Anatomy (Fig. 6-7)

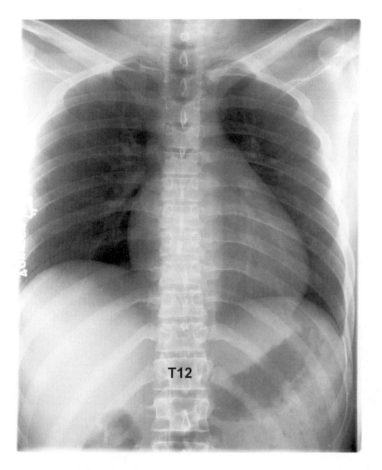

T12

**F I G U R E  6 - 7 .**  Normal thoracic spine anatomy.

## Normal Lumbar Spine Anatomy (Fig. 6-8)

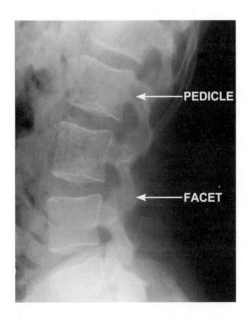

PEDICLE

FACET

**F I G U R E  6 - 8 .**  Normal lumbar spine anatomy.

### Jefferson Fracture

***LOCATION***

Burst fracture of the ring of C1.

***CAUSE***

Compression injury to the head.

***IMAGING FINDINGS***

- **Plain film open mouth view**: Lateral masses of C1 are outwardly displaced beyond the margins of the C2 vertebral body (Fig. 6-9).
- **CT**: Axial view shows the extent of the fracture throughout the ring of C1.

Patients with a Jefferson fracture frequently complain of neck pain without neurologic symptoms.

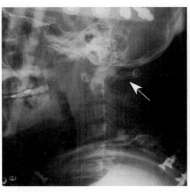 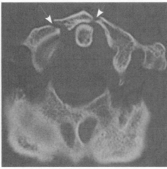 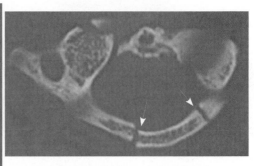

**FIGURE 6-9. Jefferson fracture on plain radiograph (left) and CT (right).**

## Dens (Odontoid) Fracture

### LOCATION

May involve the tip, base, or extend into the body of C2

### CAUSE

Flexion or extension injury that causes injury to the odontoid

### IMAGING FINDINGS

Plain film/CT findings (Fig. 6-10):

- Type I: Fracture involving the tip of the dens
- Type II: Transverse fracture involving the base of the dens
- Type III: Fracture extending into the body of C2

*Odontoid fracture:*
- Type II is the most common type of dens fracture.
- Because the type II fracture is in the axial plane, an axial CT might miss this, and coronal and sagittal reformations should be obtained.

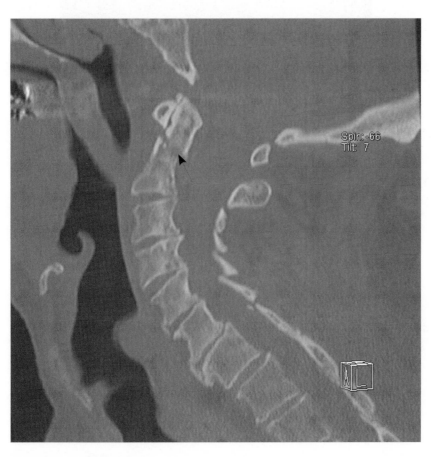

**FIGURE 6-10. Odontoid fracture.**

### Hangman's Fracture

#### LOCATION

Posterior element of C2, specifically the pars interarticularis

#### CAUSE

Caused by hyperextension injuries

#### IMAGING FINDINGS

- **Plain films:** Fracture through the bilateral pars interarticularis best seen on the lateral view just posterior the C2 vertebral body (Fig. 6-11).
- **CT:** The above findings are best seen on the sagittal view.

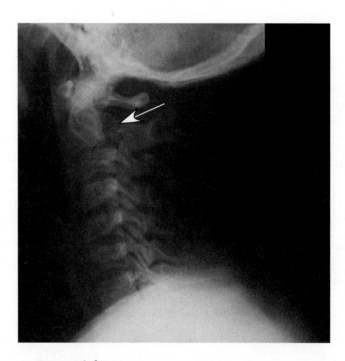

**FIGURE 6-11. Hangman's fracture.**

## Bilateral Overriding Facets in the Cervical Spine

### LOCATION

Cervical spine involving the facet joints

### CAUSE

Flexion/distraction force

### IMAGING FINDINGS

- **Lateral plain film**: 50% or greater anterolisthesis of a vertebral body relative to the adjacent one with locking of the facets at this level
- **CT**: Sagittal reformatted image shows the extent of bony injury (Fig. 6-12).

There is a high association of bilateral overriding facets with quadriplegia.

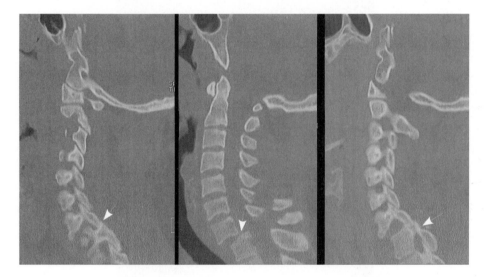

**FIGURE 6-12.** CT demonstrating marked anterolisthesis at C7–T1 of the C7 vertebral body and locked facets.

In addition, there are partially visualized spinous process fractures of C6 and C7.

### Fracture of the Posterior Spinous Process (Clay Shoveler's Fracture)

#### *LOCATION*

Posterior spinous process of C6, C7, T1, T2

#### *CAUSE*

Hyperflexion injury

#### *IMAGING FINDINGS*

Lateral plain film and sagittal CT: an oblique fracture through the posterior spinous process (Fig. 6-13).

A clay shoveler's fracture is most commonly seen at C7.

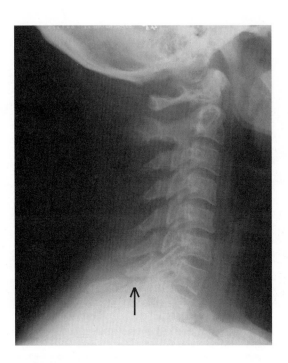

FIGURE 6-13. **Clay shoveler's fracture.**

## Hyperextension Injury

### LOCATION

Ligamentous injury in the anterior column is more common in the cervical than the thoracic spine.

### CAUSE

Backwards fall or motor vehicle accident (MVA)

### IMAGING FINDINGS

Lateral plain film and CT (Fig. 6-14):

- Widening of the anterior intervertebral disk space and facet joint
- Retrolisthesis of the upper vertebral body
- In two-thirds of patients, an avulsion fracture from the anterior inferior end plate is seen.

Retrolisthesis of the upper vertebrae may impinge on the cord and result in acute cord syndrome in hyperextension injuries.

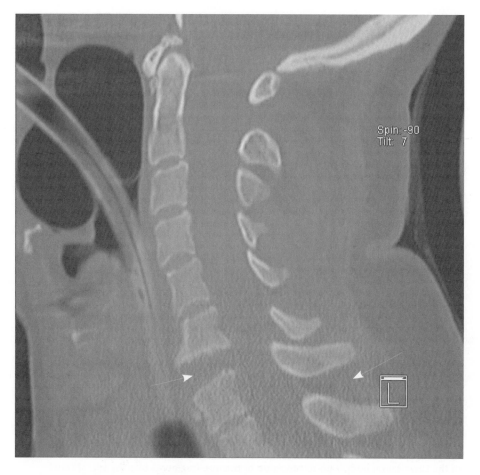

**FIGURE 6-14.** CT demonstrating widening of the anterior intervertebral disk space and spinous process between C6 and C7 is suggestive of ligamentous injury.

## Hyperflexion Injury

### LOCATION

Ligamentous injury in the posterior and middle column

If there are radiographic findings of ligamentous injury, without evidence of a fracture, an MRI should be done for further assessment.

### CAUSE

Whiplash mechanism in an MVA

### IMAGING FINDINGS

- Widening of the interspinous processes
- Kyphosis on the lateral view
- May also see anterolisthesis

## Burst Fractures

### LOCATION

In the cervical, thoracic, or lumbar spine

A burst fracture is an unstable fracture.

### CAUSE

Due to a direct axial impact injury

### IMAGING FINDINGS

- **Plain film**: May see anterior or posterior anterolisthesis of the vertebral body (Fig. 6-15)
- **CT**: Communicated fracture of the vertebral body, with retropulsion of fracture fragments into the spinal canal

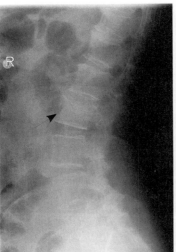
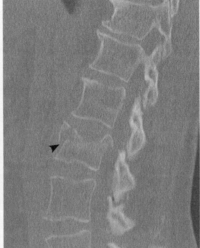
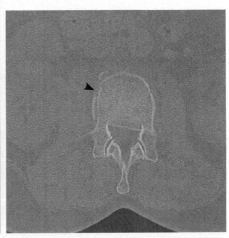

**FIGURE 6-15.** Burst fracture of the L2 vertebral body, with retropulsion of fracture fragments into the spinal canal.

## Wedge Compression Fracture

### LOCATION

Most common at the thoracolumbar junction

### CAUSE

Most commonly due to malignancy or osteoporosis

### IMAGING FINDINGS

- **Lateral plain film**: Wedge-like appearance of a vertebral body (Fig. 6-16)
- **CT**: Compression should involve no more than the anterior two-thirds of the vertebrae.
  - Wedge fractures are the most common type of lumbar fracture.
  - All patients with wedge fractures with > 50% loss of height should undergo CT to rule out burst fractures.

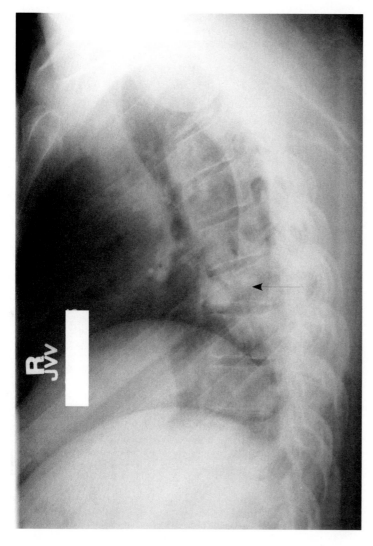

**FIGURE 6-16.** Compression fracture of the T7 vertebral body.

### Thoracic Distraction (Chance) Fracture

**LOCATION**

Usually at the thoracolumbar junction (T11–T12), but could be lower in children (L2–L4).

**CAUSE**

Hyperflexion-distraction injury involving a lap belt or an unrestrained child in an MVA.

**IMAGING FINDINGS**

- Plain films:
    - **Lateral:** Anterior compression of the vertebral body (Fig. 6-17).
    - **AP view:** May see missing spinous process.
- **CT:** Horizontal fracture through the spinous process, articulations, transverse processes, pedicles, and vertebral body.

*Chance fracture*
- More common in children than adults.
- High association with abdominal organ injury and an abdominal CT is recommended.
- Also called a seat belt fracture.

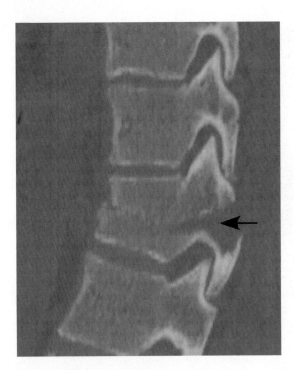

**FIGURE 6-17. Chance fracture.**

## Spondylolysis

### LOCATION

Pars interarticularis most commonly at L4 or L5.

### CAUSE

Originally thought to be congenital, but usually it is the result of trauma.

### IMAGING FINDINGS

- **Lateral plain film**: May see lucency in the pars interarticularis (Fig. 6-18).
- **Oblique plain film:** Fracture of the neck of the "Scottie dog."

If there is bilateral spondylolysis, it is called spondylolisthesis, which is anterior displacement of one vertebral body relative to the adjacent one.

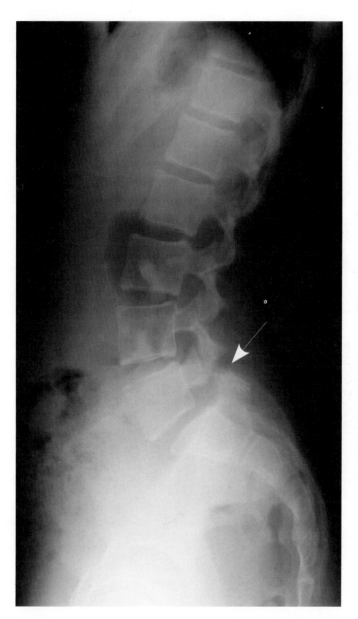

**FIGURE 6-18. Lumbar films demonstrating spondylolysis.**

Lucency through the pars interarticularis is best seen on the lateral view consistent with a pars defect.

## Multiple Myeloma

### LOCATION

Skull, axial skeleton, ribs

### CAUSE

Exact cause not clear

### IMAGING FINDINGS

Multiple lytic "punched out" lesions (Fig. 6-19)

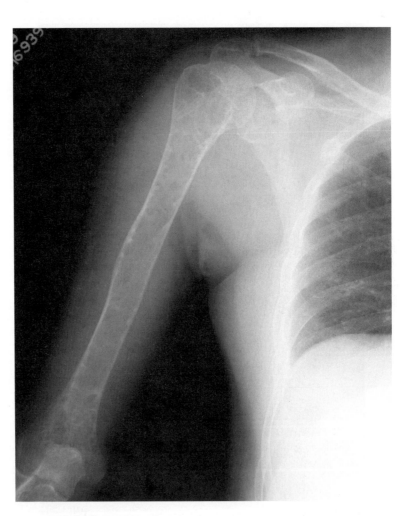

FIGURE 6-19. Plain radiograph demonstrating marked lytic changes in the humerus in a patient with multiple myeloma.

## Osteoporosis

### LOCATION

Spine and proximal extremities

### CAUSE

Postmenopausal or could be due to endocrine disorders such as hyperparathyroidism, hyperthyroidism, hypogonadism, and hypercortisolemia

### IMAGING FINDINGS:

- **Plain film:** Biconcave and end plate compression of vertebral bodies (fish vertebrae) (Fig. 6-20)
- Thin cortical bone
- **DEXA:** Lumbar spine, femoral neck, and wrists are evaluated, and T-score should be < –2.5.

- Osteoporosis is a decrease in bone mass.
- In DEXA scan, bone density is compared to a normal 30 year old (T- score).

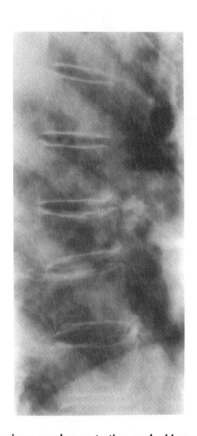

**FIGURE 6-20.** Lumbar spine x-ray demonstrating marked loss of calcification in spine, consistent with osteoporosis.

(Reproduced, with permission, from Wilson F, Lin PP: *General Orthopedics.* New York: McGraw-Hill, 1996: Figure 16.6.)

## Degenerative Changes in Spine

### LOCATION

Cervical, thoracic, and lumbar spine

### CAUSE

Degenerative

### IMAGING FINDING (FIG. 6-21)

- Disk space narrowing
- Increased density of the vertebral body end plates
- Hypertrophic changes throughout spine

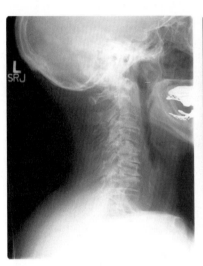
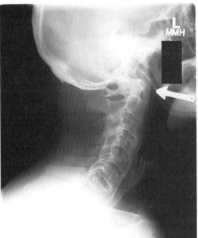
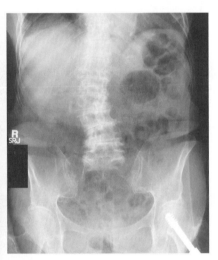

**FIGURE 6-21.** Several plain radiograph examples of severe degenerative changes in the cervical and thoracic spine. In the cervical spine films, note multilevel disk space narrowing, hypertrophic changes, and facet arthropathy.

## Ankylosing Spondylitis

### LOCATION

Spine and sacroiliac joints

### CAUSE

Autoimmune disease associated with HLA B27

### IMAGING FINDINGS (FIG. 6-22)

- **Lateral plain film**: Smooth symmetric syndesmophytes referred to as "bamboo spine"
- **AP plain film**: Fusion of the sacroiliac joints

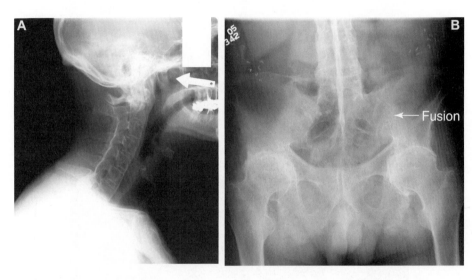

**FIGURE 6-22. Plain radiographs demonstrating changes consistent with ankylosing spondylitis.**

Note "bamboo spine" cervical spine (A), and lumbar spine film and fusion of the sacroiliac joints (B).

### Sacralization of L5

***LOCATION***

L5 and the sacrum

***CAUSE***

Normal variant

***IMAGING FINDINGS***

Unilateral or bilateral partial fusion of L5 with the sacrum (Fig. 6-23)

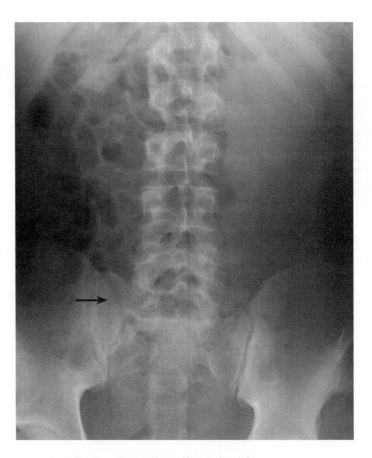

**FIGURE 6-23. Sacralization of L5 unilaterally, on the right.**

## Normal Shoulder (Fig. 6-24)

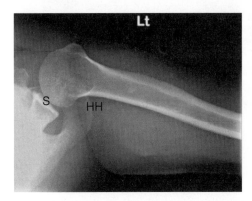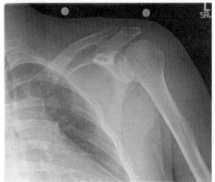

**FIGURE 6-24.** Normal axillary view (left) and AP view (right) of the left shoulder.

## Shoulder Dislocation

### LOCATION

Glenohumeral joint

### CAUSE

- Anterior dislocations are usually due to falls.
- Posterior dislocations usually due to seizures, electronconvulsive therapy, or falls.

### IMAGING FINDINGS

- **Anterior dislocation**: Humeral head lies inferior and medial to the glenohumeral joint (Fig. 6-25).
- **Posterior dislocation**: Humeral head lies posterior and superior to the glenohumeral joint (Fig. 6-26).

- Anterior dislocations are much more common than posterior dislocations.
- Anterior dislocation is associated with:
  - **Hill-Sachs fracture**: Posterior lateral impaction fracture of the humeral head.
  - **Bankart fracture**: Fracture of the glenoid labrum.

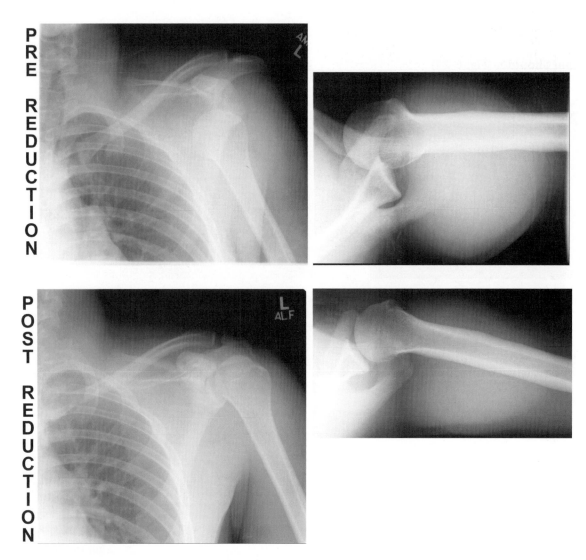

**FIGURE 6-25.** Anterior dislocation of the right shoulder with anteromedial displacement of the humerus.

Postreduction films in the same patient demonstrate normal alignment; however, there is also a resultant Hill-Sachs impaction fracture.

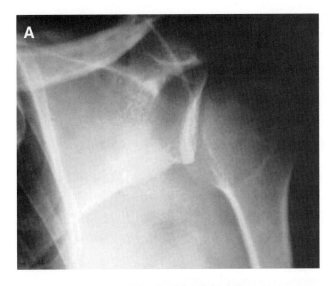
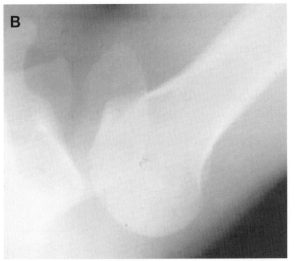

**FIGURE 6-26.** Posterior shoulder dislocation.

(A) AP view; (B) axillary view.

### Humeral Head Fracture

***LOCATION***

Proximal aspect of the humerus

***CAUSE***

Usually due to a fall

***IMAGING FINDINGS***

- **AP axillary view:** Linear or comminuted fracture through the humeral head (Fig. 6-27)
- **CT:** Shows extent of fracture and articular involvement

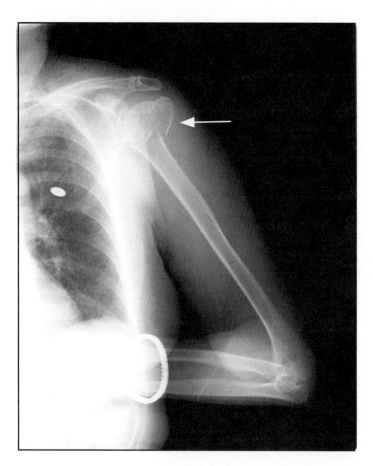

**FIGURE 6-27. Comminuted impacted fracture involving the left humeral head and neck.**

Note superolateral displacement of the greater tuberosity fragments.

## Clavicle Fracture

### LOCATION

Most commonly (80%) occurs in the middle third of the clavicle

### CAUSE

Usually results from direct injury to the shoulder

### IMAGING FINDINGS

**Routine AP x-ray**: Lucency through the clavicle which may result in a non-displaced, displaced, or communited fracture (Fig. 6-28).

In children, the clavicle is the most common fracture site in the body.

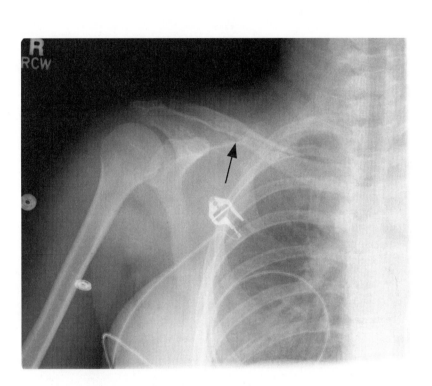

FIGURE 6-28. **Oblique minimally displaced midclavicle fracture.**

## Acromioclavicular (AC) Separation

### LOCATION

AC joint

### CAUSE

Fall injuring the AC joint region of the shoulder

### IMAGING FINDINGS

- **Routine clavicle x-ray:**
  - Type I: Due to a sprain, few ligaments torn
  - Type II: Due to rupture of the capsule and AC ligaments (Fig. 6-29)
  - Type III: Due to rupture of the AC and coracoclavicular (CC) ligaments (Fig. 6-29)

Type I and II AC separation injuries are usually managed conservatively. Type III is typically managed surgically.

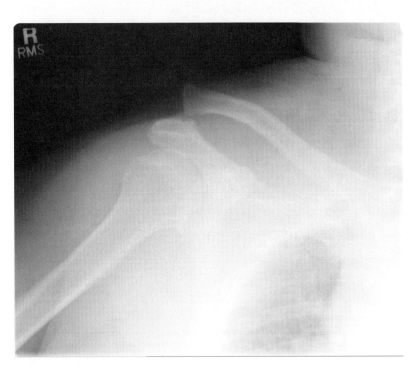

**FIGURE 6-29.** Type III separation of the AC joint with widening of the CC (white arrow) and AC (black arrow) joint spaces.

## Scapula Fracture

### LOCATION

Body, neck, spine, acromion, glenoid, or coracoid fracture

### CAUSE

Fall or MVA

### IMAGING FINDINGS

Fracture lucency through the scapula, most common in the body and spine of the scapula (Fig. 6-30)

More than 80% of scapula fractures are associated with trauma to the chest wall, lungs, and shoulder.

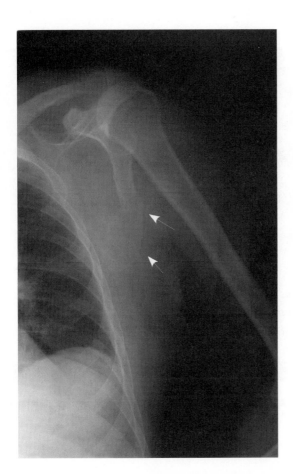

**FIGURE 6-30.** Comminuted minimally displaced fracture of the body of the left scapula.

## Os Acromiale

### *LOCATION*

Center of the acromion

### *CAUSE*

Secondary ossification center that normally fuses by age 24

### *IMAGING FINDINGS*

Well-corticated bony fragment at the anterior end of the acromion (Fig. 6-31).

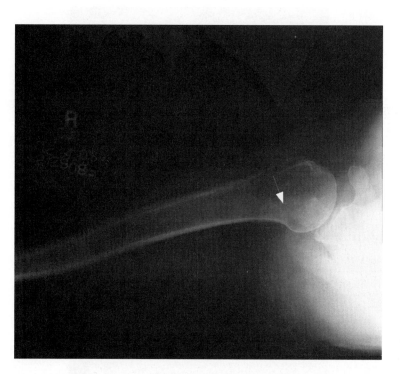

**FIGURE 6-31. Axillary view demonstrates a normal variant os acromiale.**

## Degenerative Arthritis of the Shoulder

### LOCATION

Glenohumeral joint

### CAUSE

Degenerative, could also be from rotator cuff tears

### IMAGING FINDINGS

Plain film (Fig. 6-32):

- Calcification of tendons
- Narrowing of the glenohumeral joint space
- Hypertrophic changes surrounding the joint
- Flattening of the humeral head

Rotator cuff tears are best seen with MRI.

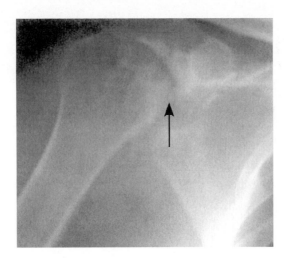

**FIGURE 6-32. X-ray of the right shoulder demonstrates superior subluxation of the humeral head, severe joint space narrowing (arrow), and periarticular osteoporosis, consistent with advanced degenerative joint disease.**

HIGH-YIELD FACTS

Musculoskeletal Radiology

**Normal Elbow Anatomy (Fig. 6-33)**

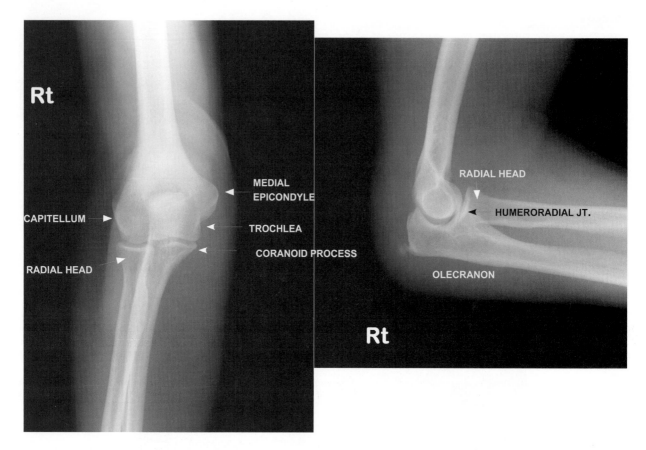

FIGURE 6-33. **Normal elbow anatomy.**

## Radial Head Fracture

### *LOCATION*

Radial head

### *CAUSE*

Fall on outstretched hand

### *IMAGING FINDINGS (FIG. 6-34)*

X-ray:

- May see a minimally or nondisplaced fracture of the radial head
- Key imaging finding is displacement of the anterior and/or posterior fat pads due to intraarticular extension of the fracture causing hemarthrosis.
- A radial head fracture is the most common fracture in the elbow of an adult.
- A radial head fracture may not be seen on AP and lateral views; an oblique view should be ordered if the patient is tender.
- "Sail sign" is anterior displacement of the anterior fat pad due to effusion of hemorrhage.
- You should never see the posterior fat pad!

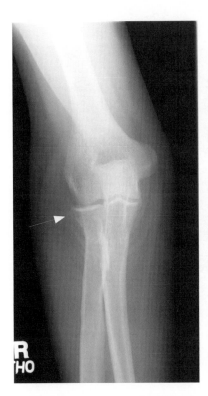
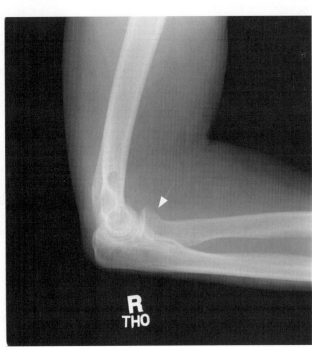

FIGURE 6-34. **Minimally displaced intra-articular fracture of the radial head.**

Supracondylar fractures
are usually seen in children
aged 9 to 12 years.

## Supracondylar Fracture

### *LOCATION*

Distal humerus

### *CAUSE*

Fall on outstretched hand

### *IMAGING FINDINGS*

**AP and lateral views:** May see a nondisplaced or displaced fracture through the supracondylar region of the humerus (Fig. 6-35).

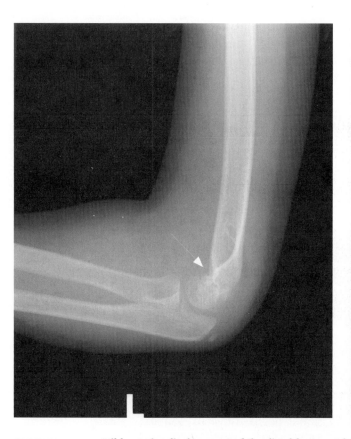
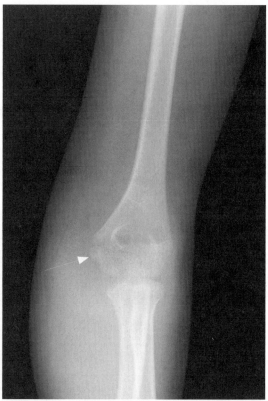

**FIGURE 6-35.** Mild anterior displacement of the distal fragment fracture of a supracondylar fracture.

## Normal Forearm Anatomy (Fig. 6-36)

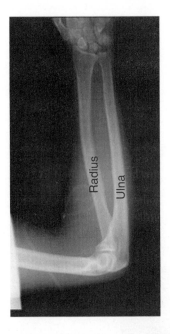

**FIGURE 6-36.** Normal forearm anatomy.

## Normal Wrist Anatomy (Figs. 6-37 and 6-38)

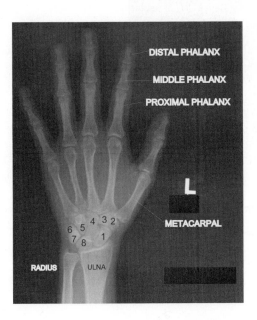

**FIGURE 6-37.** Normal hand and wrist anatomy.

Note numbered carpal bones: 1, scaphoid; 2, trapezium; 3, trapezoid; 4, capitate; 5, hamate; 6, triquetrium; 7, pisiform; 8, lunate.

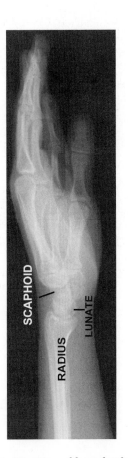

**FIGURE 6-38.** Normal lateral wrist anatomy.

### Night Stick Fracture

#### LOCATION

Mid ulna

#### CAUSE

- By crossing the arm in front of the face for protection. This is how the fracture got its name.
- Direct injury to the ulna.

#### IMAGING FINDINGS

**AP and lateral view:** Forearm: Simple fracture through the middle of the ulna (Fig. 6-39).

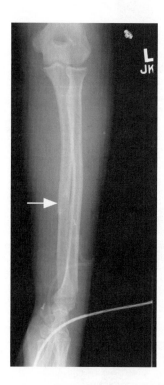

**FIGURE 6-39.** Oblique fracture through the shaft of the ulna with minimal displacement; also known as a nightstick fracture.

## Olecranon Fracture

### LOCATION

Olecranon

### CAUSE

Fall on an outstretched arm or direct trauma. Results from a sudden pull of both the triceps and brachialis muscles

### IMAGING FINDINGS (FIG. 6-40)

Two main types of fractures:

- **Comminuted**: From direct trauma to the olecranon
- **Transverse**: Due to a fall on outstretched hand with triceps contracted

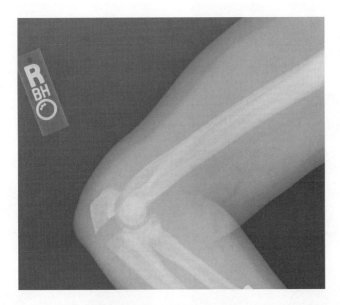

**FIGURE 6-40.** Lateral view shows a transverse intra-articular fracture of the olecranon with distraction of the proximal fracture fragment.

Olecranon fractures most commonly occur in elderly patients.

A Colles' fracture is the most common fracture of the forearm. CT may be ordered if there is a question of intra-articular extension, and for preoperative planning.

### Colles' Fracture

#### LOCATION

- Distal radius
- Ulnar styloid sometimes

#### CAUSE

Fall on an outstretched hand

#### IMAGING FINDINGS (FIG. 6-41)

- Transverse, often communicated fracture of the distal radius with dorsal angulation of the distal fracture fragment
- Associated fracture of the ulnar styloid process sometimes seen

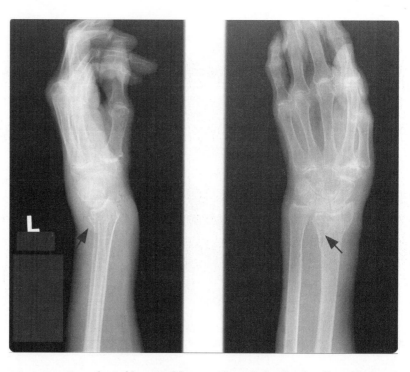

**FIGURE 6-41.** **Comminuted impacted fracture through the distal radius with dorsal angulation (single arrow) of the distal fracture fragments and intra-articular extension.**

Minimal displaced ulnar styloid fracture (double arrow).

## Scaphoid Fracture

### LOCATION

Scaphoid bone

### CAUSE

Fall on outstretched hand

### IMAGING FINDINGS

**AP, lateral, and scaphoid views:** Most are transverse fractures through the long axis of the bone (Fig. 6-42).

- The most common fracture of the carpal bones is a scaphoid fracture.
- Common complications of a scaphoid fracture are avascular necrosis and nonunion.
- An MRI, bone scan, or CT could be obtained to evaluate for an occult scaphoid fracture.

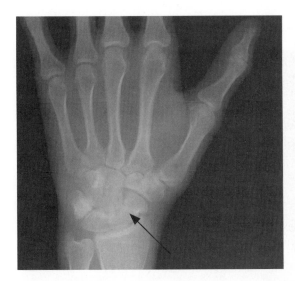
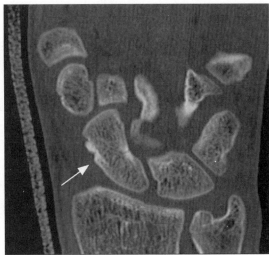

**FIGURE 6-42. Nondisplaced transverse fracture through the scaphoid waist.**

- Fourth and fifth metacarpals are most commonly injured.
- Boxer fracture: Fracture of the distal fifth metacarpal.
- Bennett fracture: Linear fracture at the base of the first metacarpal with intra-articular extension.
- Rolando fracture: Same as Bennett fracture except the fracture is comminuted.

## Metacarpal Fractures

### LOCATION

Metacarpal bones

### CAUSE

Usually direct trauma

### IMAGING FINDINGS (FIG. 6-43)

- Lucent fracture lines
- Check for intra-articular extension and associated dislocation

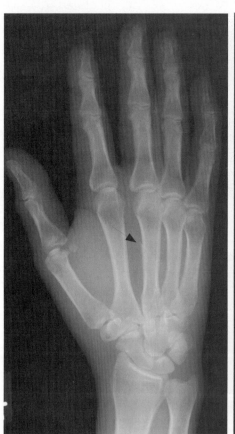
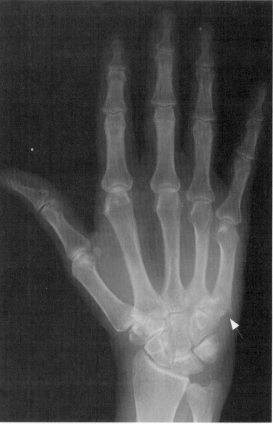

**FIGURE 6-43. Metacarpal fractures.**

(A) Oblique minimally displaced fracture through the shaft of the third metacarpal. (B) Comminuted fracture at the base of the fifth metacarpal with intra-articular extension.

## Phalangeal Fractures

### LOCATION

Proximal, middle, or distal phalanx

### CAUSE

Usually direct trauma

### IMAGING FINDINGS

- **PA and lateral views:** Simple or comminuted fracture in the proximal, middle, or distal phalanx (Fig. 6-44).
- **In children:** Salter-Harris classification is used (Fig. 7-24).

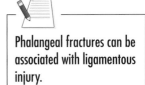

Phalangeal fractures can be associated with ligamentous injury.

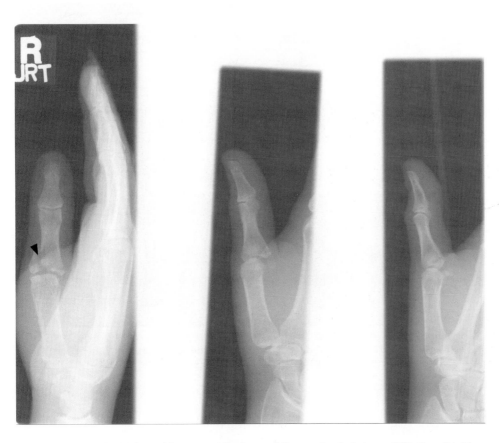

**FIGURE 6-44.** Comminuted fracture at the base of the proximal phalanx of the thumb with intra-articular extension.

### Phalangeal/Metacarpal Dislocation

#### *LOCATION*

At the IP or MCP joints of the hands

#### *CAUSE*

Trauma

#### *IMAGING FINDINGS*

Palmar or dorsal dislocation at the IP (Fig. 6-45)

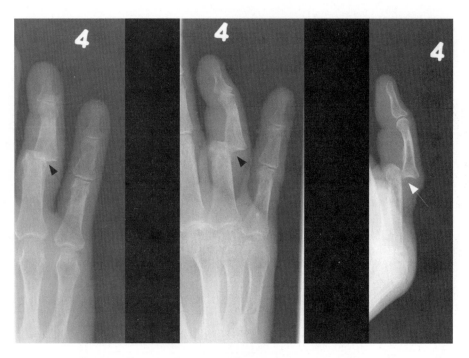

**FIGURE 6-45.** Dorsal dislocation of the proximal interphalangeal joint of the fourth digit.

### Rheumatoid Arthritis

#### LOCATION

PIP joint, MCP joint, wrists, MTP, ankles, knee, shoulders.

#### CAUSE

Autoimmune.

#### IMAGING FINDINGS

AP and lateral views of the hands (Fig. 6-46):

- **Early:** Soft tissue swelling around joints, marginal bone erosions, osteopenia around the joints
- **Late:** Diffuse osteopenia, joint subluxations, soft tissue wasting, rheumatoid nodules, ulnar deviation at the MCP joints

- **Boutonniere deformity:** Flexion in the PIP joint and hyperextension of the DIP joint
- **Swan neck deformity:** Hyperextension of the PIP joint and flexion of the DIP joint

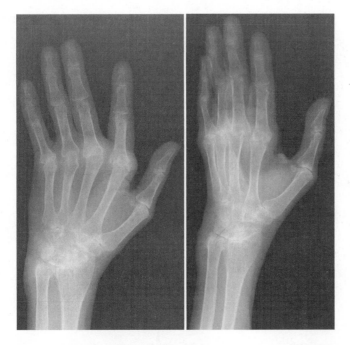

**FIGURE 6-46.** **Joint space narrowing and erosive changes at the second through fifth metacarpal phalangeal joints. Findings consistent with RA.**

## Psoriatic Arthritis

### LOCATION

Distal interphalangeal joints of the fingers and toes in an asymmetric distribution

### CAUSE

Pathogenesis of psoriatic arthritis remains unknown

### IMAGING FINDINGS

- Resorption of the tufts of the distal phalanges with malalignment and subluxation of joints known as the "opera glass hand"
- In some cases terminal phalanx may become sclerotic (ivory phalanx).
- Erosions with ill-defined margins and adjacent periosteal proliferation may lead to the characteristic "pencil in cup" deformity (Fig. 6-47).

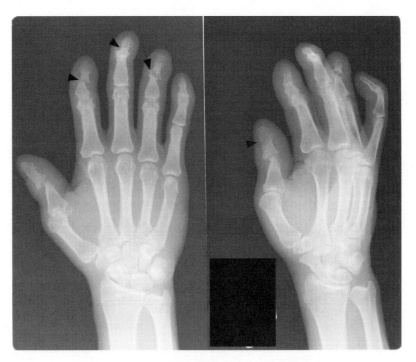

**FIGURE 6-47.** Severe erosive arthritis involving the distal hand joints. In addition, the "pencil in cup" deformity is present at the first digit.

## ▶ INCREASING FRACTURE VISIBILITY OVER TIME

### *LOCATION*

Any fracture site

### *CAUSE*

A fracture becomes more visible a week after the injury due to subsequent decalcification after the initial injury.

### *IMAGING FINDINGS*

Fracture 7 to10 days after initial injury is more apparent than on initial films.

If an x-ray is negative at the time of an injury, a repeat x-ray in 7 to 10 days could be obtained since the initial fracture may be occult.

## ▶ DISUSE OSTEOPENIA

### *LOCATION*

Any bony injury after a fracture

### *CAUSE*

Loss of calcium that occurs weeks or months after an injury due to disuse of the immobilized injured body part

### *IMAGING FINDINGS*

Demineralization of bone with loss of the trabecular pattern in a periarticular distribution in close proximity to a fracture

Musculoskeletal Radiology

## Normal Pelvis Anatomy (Fig. 6-48)

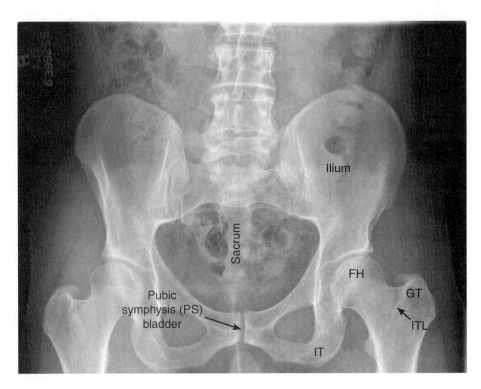

**FIGURE 6-48. Normal AP view of pelvis anatomy.**

FH, fibular head; GT, greater trochanter; IT, ischial tuberosity; ITL, intertrochanteric line

## Normal Femur Anatomy (Fig. 6-49)

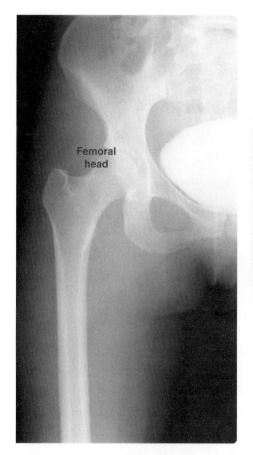
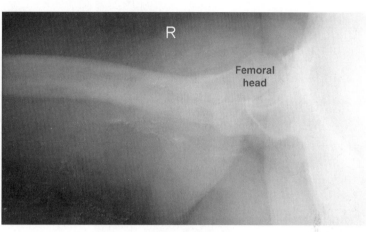

FIGURE 6-49. Normal AP and lateral views of femur anatomy.

## Normal Tibia and Fibula Anatomy (Fig. 6-50)

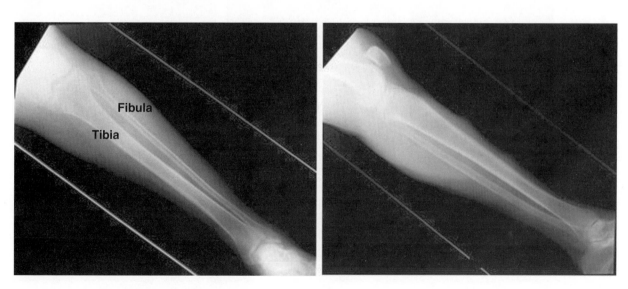

FIGURE 6-50. Normal tibia/fibula anatomy.

## Normal Knee Anatomy (Fig. 6-51)

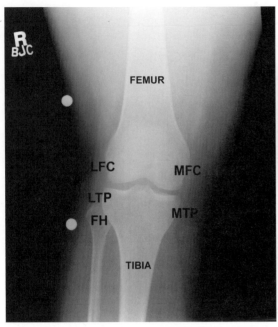
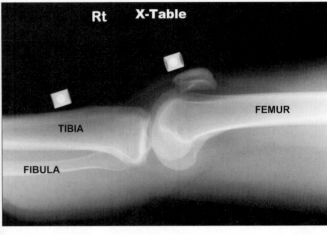

**FIGURE 6-51.** Normal knee anatomy.

LFC, lateral femoral condyle; MFC, medial femoral condyle; FH, fibular head; LTP, lateral tibial plateau; MTP, medial tibial plateau

## Normal Ankle Anatomy (Fig. 6-52)

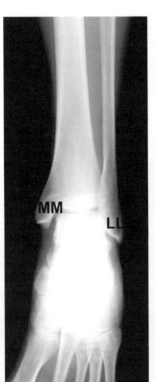
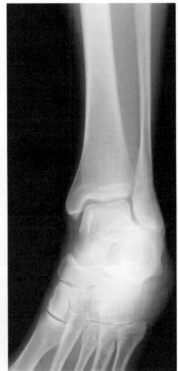
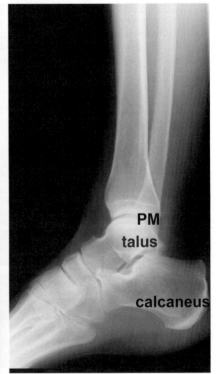

**FIGURE 6-52.** Normal ankle anatomy.

MM, medial malleolus; LM, lateral malleolus; PM, posterior malleolus

## Normal Foot Anatomy (Fig. 6-53)

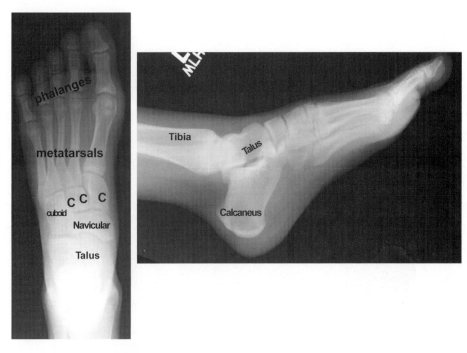

**FIGURE 6-53. Normal foot anatomy.**

C = medial, middle, and lateral cuneiform

- Posterior dislocation accounts for 90% of hip dislocations.
- Due to the risk of avascular necrosis of an unreduced hip, dislocation is an orthopedic emergency.

### Posterior Hip Dislocation

#### LOCATION

Hip joint

#### CAUSE

Patient's leg is in a flexed and adducted position and strikes the dashboard in an MVA.

#### IMAGING FINDINGS

The femoral head is displaced superior and laterally. Femoral head is located posterior to the acetabulum (Fig. 6-54).

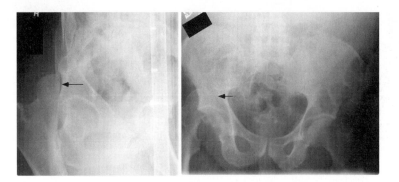

**FIGURE 6-54. Posterior hip dislocation.**

## Anterior Hip Dislocation (Fig. 6-55)

### LOCATION

Hip joint

### CAUSE

Involves forced abduction and external rotation

### IMAGING FINDINGS

- The femoral head is displaced inferiorly and medially and usually overlies the obturator ring.
- Femoral head is located anterior to the acetabulum.

CT scan should be performed for all hip dislocations to look for bony fragments or femoral/acetabular fractures, which occurs in 10% of all hip dislocations.

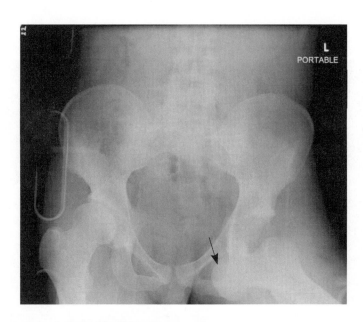

**FIGURE 6-55. Anterior hip dislocation.**

Malignant degeneration occurs in up to 10% of patients with osteosarcoma or fibrosarcoma.

## Paget's Disease

### LOCATION

Most common sites involved are the axial skeleton, femur, and tibia.

### CAUSE

Etiology unknown.

### IMAGING FINDINGS (FIG. 6-56)

- Thickening of the iliopectineal line
- Coarsening of the trabecula
- Thickened cortex
- "Blade of grass" appearance of the long bones
- Increased size of the involved bone

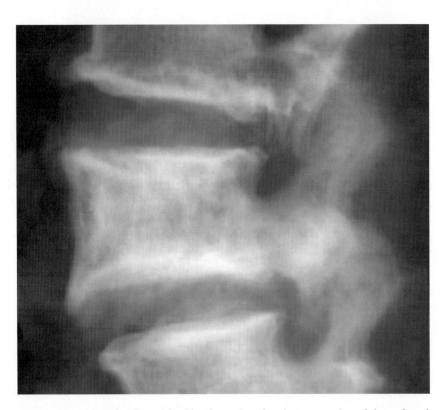

**FIGURE 6-56.** Lateral radiograph of lumbar spine showing coarsening of the trabecula, increased size of the vertebral body, and thickening of the cortex, which is classic for Paget's disease.

## Osteopetrosis

### LOCATION

All bones of the body

### CAUSE

Problems with osteoclasts

Patients with osteopetrosis are extremely prone to fractures.

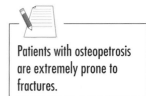

### IMAGING FINDINGS (FIG. 6-57)

- Extremely dense bones
- May see "bone within a bone appearance" on lateral x-ray

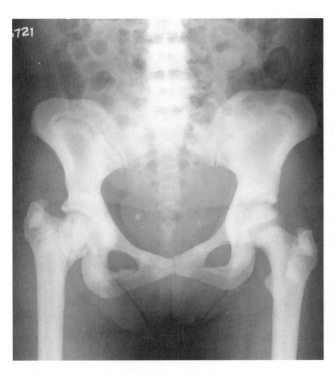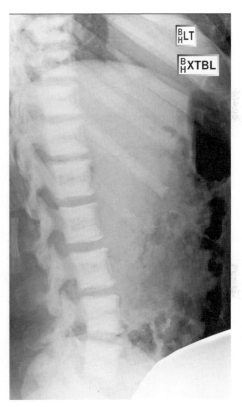

**FIGURE 6-57.** Diffuse increase in density of bones consistent with osteopetrosis.

In addition, the thoracic spine shows the classic bone within a bone appearance (arrow).

Osteogenic sarcoma is the most frequent type of bone tumor and is most common between the ages of 15 and 25 years.

## Osteosarcoma

### LOCATION

Metaphyses of long bones (commonly femur) are the most common site; flat bones account for a very small percentage, and among these the ilium is the most common.

### CAUSE

May be due to malignant degeneration of Paget's disease or due to radiation

### IMAGING FINDINGS

- Destructive appearing, lytic and/or blastic mass
- Periosteal reaction may be laminated or spiculated with so-called "sunburst" appearance (see Figure 6-58).
- Variable amount of calcification in the soft tissues.
- Codman's triangle is due to elevation of the periosteum from the cortical bone.

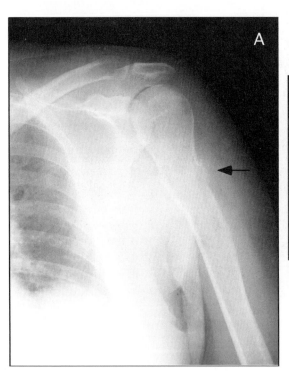
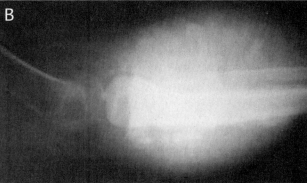

**FIGURE 6-58. Osteosarcoma.**

(A) Mixed lytic and sclerotic lesion in the proximal femur with periosteal new bone formation, and soft tissue swelling.
(B) X-ray of the extremity showing typical sunburst appearance in osteosarcoma.

## Bone Metastasis

### LOCATION

Proximal long bones and axial skeleton

### CAUSE

- **Lytic (lucent) metastasis:** Breast, lung, thyroid, GI tumors, and melanoma
- **Blastic (sclerotic) metastasis:** Prostate, breast, lung, and carcinoid

### IMAGING FINDINGS

Lytic, sclerotic, or mixed lesions (Fig. 6-59)

In most cases, the best screening technique is a radionuclide bone scan to detect bone metastasis.

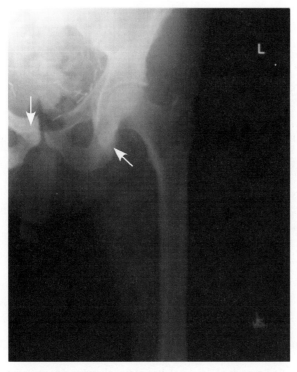

**FIGURE 6-59.** Pelvic x-ray depicting multiple sclerotic appearing bone metastasis seen in a patient with prostate cancer.

Various abnormal changes may complicate degenerative joint disease, the most important being joint malalignment, subluxation, ankylosis, and intra-articular loose bodies.

### Osteoarthritis

#### LOCATION

At the knee joint

#### CAUSE

Degenerative

#### IMAGING FINDINGS (FIG. 6-60)

- Joint space narrowing and sclerosis of the medial and lateral compartments
- Hypertrophic changes are often seen

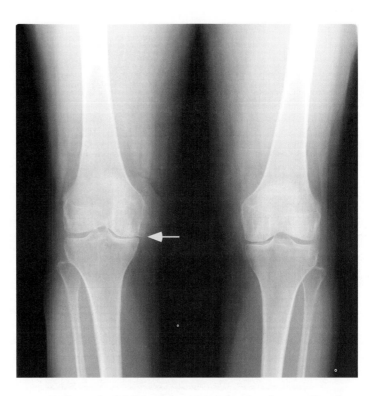

FIGURE 6-60. Radiograph of bilateral knee joint showing degenerative changes with medial compartment narrowing, more marked on the right.

## Septic Arthritis

### LOCATION

Most commonly involved joints in septic arthritis is the knee (50%), followed by hip (20%), shoulder (8%), ankle (7%), and wrists (7%).

### CAUSE

Organisms invade the joint directly, by contiguous spread, or the bloodstream.

### IMAGING FINDINGS

- Periarticular soft tissue swelling, widening of the joint space
- In later stages may see joint space narrowing and bony erosions

Ultrasound can be used to evaluate for an effusion and guide treatment.

## Femoral Neck Fracture

### LOCATION

- Neck of the femur
- Further divided into subcapital, transcervical, and base of the neck

### CAUSE

Usually trauma or fall.

### IMAGING FINDINGS

- **Subcapital**: Most proximal portion of the neck, adjacent to the femoral head (Fig. 6-61)
- **Transcervical**: Fracture through the middle of the neck
- **Base of the neck**: Most distal portion of the neck just proximal to the greater and lesser trochanter

Femoral neck fractures:
- Subcapital fracture is the most common type.
- Occur most commonly in elderly females.
- Avascular necrosis is a common complication.

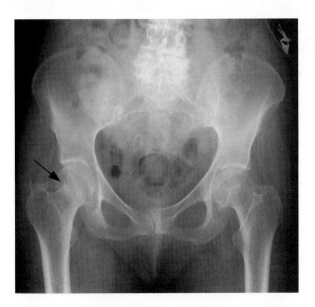

**FIGURE 6-61. Femoral neck fracture. Subcapital fracture through the right femoral neck.**

### Intertrochanteric Fracture (Fig. 6-62)

*LOCATION*

Between the greater and lesser trochanters

*CAUSE*

Usually secondary to fall

*IMAGING FINDINGS*

- Fracture extending from the greater to the lesser trochanter
- There may also be multiple fracture fragments

Intertrochanteric fractures typically occur in elderly patients.

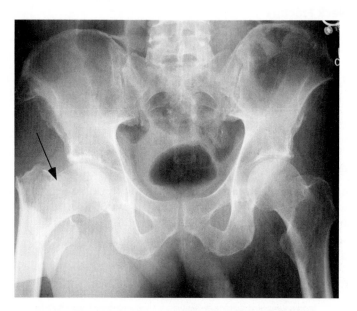

**FIGURE 6-62. Intertrochanteric fracture.** Oblique intertrochanteric fracture of the right femur with superior displacement of the distal fracture fragment relative to the femoral head.

## Fibrous Cortical Defect

### LOCATION

Distal femur, distal tibia

### CAUSE

Developmental

### IMAGING FINDINGS

Well-circumscribed lytic defect with sclerotic margins in the metaphysis of long bones (Fig. 6-63)

A fibrous cortical defect is a benign lesion and requires no treatment unless there is a fracture.

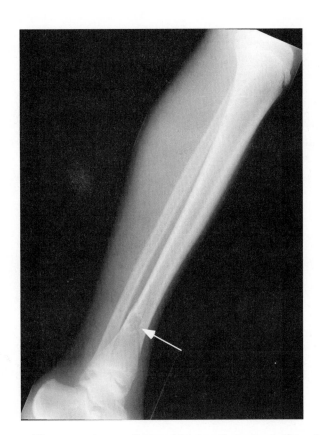

**FIGURE 6-63.** Oblique complex nondisplaced fracture that extends through a benign fibrous cortical defect.

### Knee Effusion

#### LOCATION

Just above the patella; best seen on the lateral view

#### CAUSE

Trauma or degenerative changes

#### IMAGING FINDINGS

Increased opacity on the lateral view just superior to the patella (Fig. 6-64)

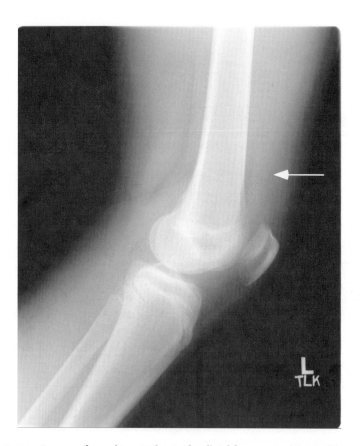

**FIGURE 6-64.** Increased opacity anterior to the distal femur, consistent with an effusion.

## Patella Fracture

### LOCATION

Patella

### CAUSE

Usually caused by direct trauma to the patella

### IMAGING FINDINGS (FIG. 6-65)

- Sharp lucent lines through the patella
- Look for associated soft tissue swelling

Do not mistake patella fracture for a bipartite patella.

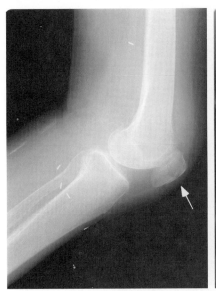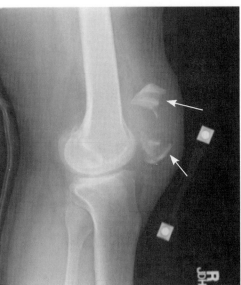

FIGURE 6-65. Nondisplaced comminuted fracture of the patella.

### Tibia-Fibula Shaft Fractures

#### *LOCATION*

Shaft of the tibia and/or fibula or both

#### *CAUSE*

Usually trauma

#### *IMAGING FINDINGS*

Fracture through the tibia and/or fibula which may be displaced and angulated (Fig. 6-66).

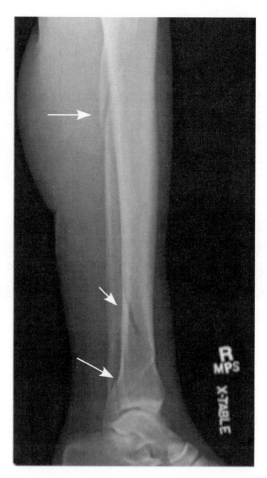

**FIGURE 6-66. Oblique fracture through the proximal fibula, distal tibia, and posterior malleolus.**

## Tibial Plateau Fractures

### *LOCATION*

Tibial plateau

### *CAUSE*

MVAs or fall

### *IMAGING FINDINGS (FIG. 6-67)*

- **Elderly**: Sclerosis and depression of the tibial plateau
- **Young adults**: Lucent fracture line through the tibial plateau

- The most common fracture of the proximal tibia is the tibial plateau fracture.
- AP and lateral x-rays are usually diagnostic of a tibial plateau fracture.

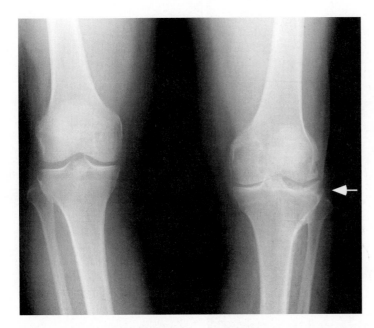

**FIGURE 6-67.** Left lateral tibial plateau fracture with depression of the articular surface.

- Most common fracture of the ankle is the medial or lateral malleolus fracture.
- If the posterior malleolus is fractured, there is usually an associated medial or lateral malleolar fracture.
- Described as a bimalleolar fracture if it involves both the medial and lateral malleolus
- Described as a trimalleolar fracture if it involves the posterior, medial, and lateral malleolus

## Malleolar Fractures

### LOCATION

Medial, lateral, or posterior malleolus

### CAUSE

Usually trauma

### IMAGING FINDINGS

Fractures through the medial and/or lateral and posterior malleolus (Fig. 6-68)

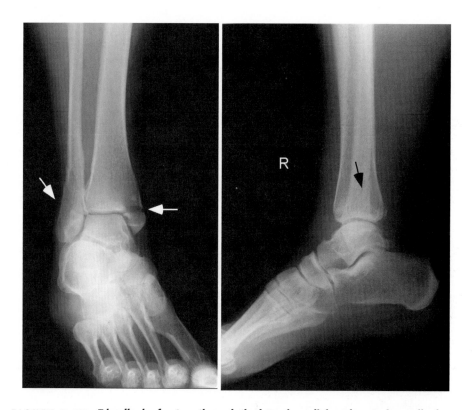

**FIGURE 6-68. Trimalleolar fracture through the lateral, medial, and posterior malleolus.**

## Ligamentous Injury

### LOCATION

- **Medially:** Deltoid ligament
- **Laterally:** Anterior and posterior talofibular and calcaneofibular joint

### CAUSE

Usually trauma

### IMAGING FINDINGS

**Stress views:** Shows abnormal widening of the ankle joint

## Jones Fracture

### LOCATION

Base of the fifth metatarsal

### CAUSE

Inversion injury to the foot

### IMAGING FINDINGS

Transverse fracture through the base of the fifth metatarsal (Fig. 6-69)

- Lateral ligament is the most commonly injured.
- Stress view x-rays are taken while the ankle is turned side to side.

Do not mistake a normal apophysis, which is parallel to the long axis of the metatarsal, for a Jones fracture!

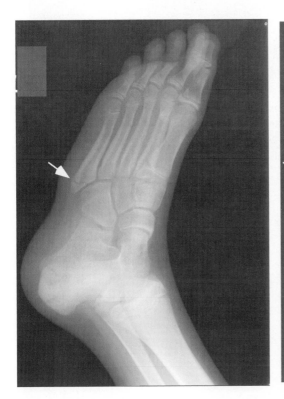
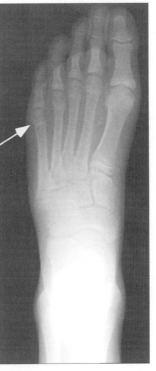

**FIGURE 6-69.** **Transverse fracture through the base of the fifth metatarsal.**

### Lisfranc Fracture/Dislocation

#### LOCATION

Tarsal-metatarsal joints of the second through fifth metatarsals

#### CAUSE

Direct trauma

#### IMAGING FINDINGS

Fracture and lateral dislocation of the second, third, fourth, and fifth metatarsal. Up to 20% of Lisfranc fractures/dislocations are missed on x-rays. (Fig. 6-70).

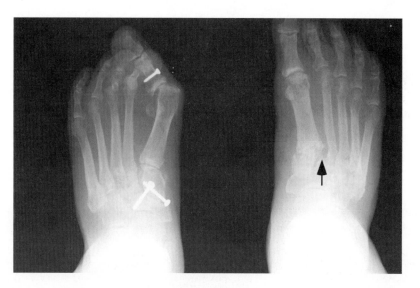

**FIGURE 6-70.** The tarsal-metatarsal joints of the second through fifth metatarsals of the right midfoot are fractured and laterally dislocated consistent with a Lisfranc fracture/dislocation.

## Stress (March) Fractures

### LOCATION

Second metatarsal is the most common location, followed closely by the third metatarsal.

### CAUSE

- Continued stress to an otherwise normal bone
- Seen most often in military personnel who march long distances

### IMAGING FINDINGS

Sclerosis, periosteal reaction usually in the distal metatarsals

## Osteomyelitis

### LOCATION

Most common in the toes

### CAUSE

Occurs when infection occurs in a bone, or spreads from another organ.

### IMAGING FINDINGS

Soft tissue swelling (see Fig. 6-71), periosteal reaction, bony destruction, and loss of trabecular pattern

Initial x-ray is usually normal, but becomes positive 2 to 14 days later.

- Osteomyelitis may be present despite a normal x-ray. So if clinical suspicion is high, an MRI would be useful for further evaluation.
- In cellulitis there should be no bony changes, only soft tissue swelling.

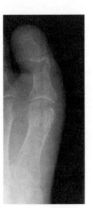

**FIGURE 6-71.** Soft tissue swelling about the left first toe in a patient with known osteomyelitis.

HIGH-YIELD FACTS

Musculoskeletal Radiology

# Pediatric Radiology

### Tuberous Sclerosis

#### CAUSE

Autosomal dominant genetic disorder that causes benign tumors to grow in the brain and on other vital organs such as the kidneys, heart, eyes, lungs, and skin.

#### IMAGING FINDINGS

CT scan reveals small, sometimes calcified nodular lesions (tubers) in paraventricular distribution (Fig. 7-1).

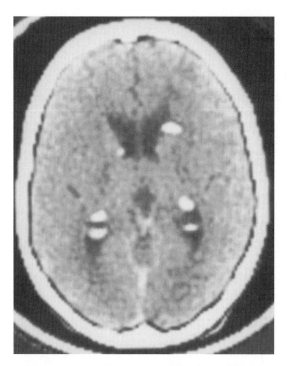

**FIGURE 7-1. Noncontrast CT of brain depicting tuberous sclerosis.**

Triad of tuberous sclerosis:
- Facial nevus (adenoma sebaceum)
- Seizures
- Mental deficiency

## Dandy-Walker Syndrome

### CAUSE

Obstruction at the level of foramina of Luschka and Magendie.

### IMAGING FINDINGS

- Cystic dilatation of the fourth ventricle with varying degree of hypoplasia or aplasia of cerebellar vermis. CT or MRI is test of choice (Fig. 7-2).
- Characteristic findings include hypoplastic/absent cerebellar vermis and hemispheres, large fluid-filled fourth ventricle communicating with a posterior fossa cyst, and a high tentorium.
- Needs to be differentiated from mega cisterna magna, which has a normal cerebellar vermis

Majority of patients with Dandy-Walker malformation develop postnatal hydrocephalus.

The most common accompanying cerebral anomaly in Dandy-Walker malformation is agenesis/hypogenesis of the corpus callosum.

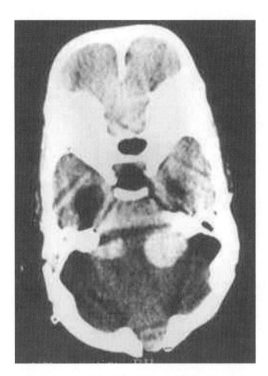

**FIGURE 7-2.** Noncontrast brain CT depicting Dandy-Walker malformation.

There is a large posterior fossa cyst of CSF density, communicating with the fourth ventricle. Also noted is an occipital defect due to associated encephalocele.

### Neurologic Neoplasms

- Most common intracranial pediatric neoplasms are astrocytoma, medulloblastoma, ependymomas, and craniopharyngiomas.
- Astrocytomas are usually cerebellar in location. These may be solid or cystic. Cystic tumors have an enhancing mural nodule.

▶ CHEST

### Croup (Laryngotracheobronchitis)

- Important infectious cause of airway obstruction in young children.
- Most common etiology is viral.
- Radiological diagnosis: X-ray of neck soft tissue reveals subglottic narrowing known as "steeple" sign (Fig. 7-3).

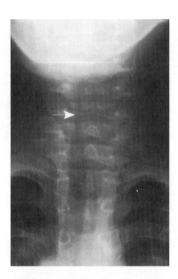

**FIGURE 7-3. Steeple sign of laryngotracheobronchitis.**

## Epiglottitis

- Medical emergency that needs immediate treatment
- Radiological diagnosis: Swollen epiglottis on lateral view, known as the "thumb" sign (Fig. 7-4)

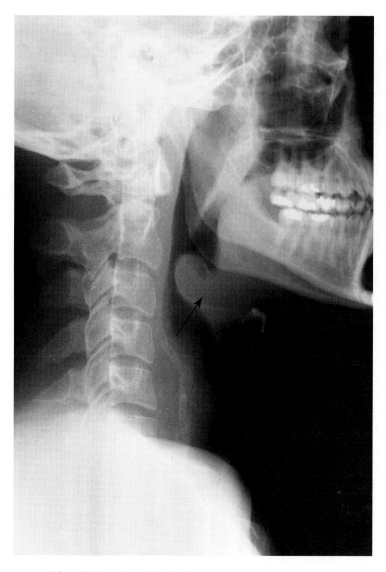

**FIGURE 7-4.** *"Thumb" sign of epiglottitis (arrow).*

## Pneumonia

### IMAGING FINDINGS

- Look for air bronchograms. Localize the segment involved.
- For right upper lobe involvement, rule out thymic shadow vs. infiltrate (Fig. 7-5).

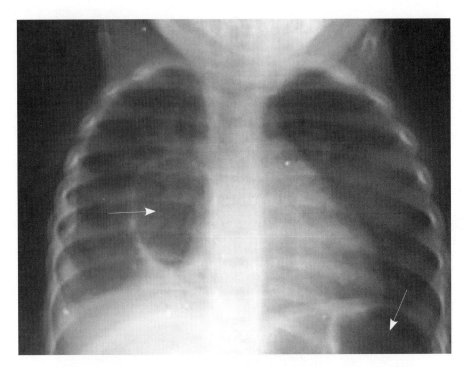

**FIGURE 7-5. Pneumonia in a child. Note typical pneumatocoeles (arrows) seen with staphylococcal infection.**

## Peritonsillar/Retropharyngeal Abscess

- Complication of upper respiratory tract infection.
- Lateral neck X-ray is preliminary test. Not very sensitive. Findings are dependent on the technique and positioning of the child.
- Diagnostic findings are prevertebral soft tissue thickness > 7 mm at C2, and 14 mm at C6. One may also find gas-fluid levels or foreign body in soft tissue (Fig. 7-6).

Contrast-enhanced CT scan is better for retropharyngeal abscess evaluation. It can clearly delineate the abscess as a hypodense area with rim enhancement. It also gives details regarding exact extent and relationship with adjoining structures.

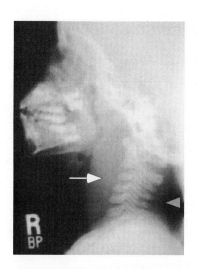

**FIGURE 7-6. Lateral radiograpah of the soft tissue of the neck.**

Note the large amount of prevertebral edema (solid arrow), and the collection of air (dashed arrow). Findings are consistent with retropharyngeal abscess. (Photo courtesy Dr. Gregory J. Schears.)

## Foreign Bodies

### CAUSE

Most commonly ingested foreign body in children is a coin.

### IMAGING FINDINGS

- Coin within esophagus appears flat on an AP view and on edge in the lateral view (Fig. 7-7).
- Most common complication is from foreign body impaction within the esophagus.
- Children with known anomalies have impactions commonly at the known anomalous sites.

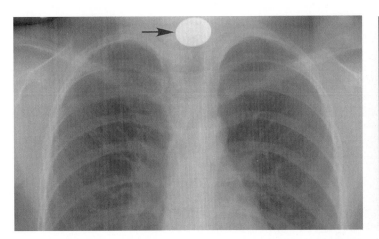 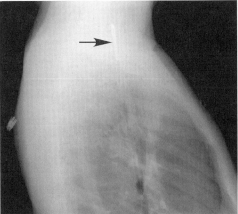

**FIGURE 7-7. AP and lateral views demonstrating a coin in the esophagus.**

A coin in the trachea would be present in the opposite manner—the coin would be seen on edge in the lateral view, and flat on the AP view.

## Tetralogy of Fallot

### CAUSE

Cyanotic congenital anomaly

### IMAGING FINDINGS

Classic CXR finding: Boot-shaped heart. Radiological features include normal-size heart, concave main pulmonary artery shadow, and reduced pulmonary vascularity (Fig. 7-8).

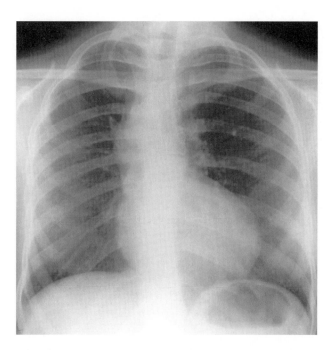

**FIGURE 7-8.** **CXR demonstrating decreased pulmonary vascularity, normal cardiac size, concave main pulmonary artery segment, and right aortic arch.**

Note boot-shaped heart (*Coeur en sabot*) secondary to the uplifting of the cardiac apex from right ventricular hypertrophy and the concave main pulmonary artery segment with decreased pulmonary vascularity.

### Transposition of the Great Arteries (TGA): Egg-Shaped Heart

#### CAUSE

Abnormal division of bulbar trunk during embryogenesis leads to opposite origins of aorta and pulmonary artery. Aorta arises from morphological right ventricle, and pulmonary artery from morphological left ventricle.

#### CXR FINDINGS

Will include cardiomegaly and the classical sign, "egg on side" appearance (Fig. 7-9).

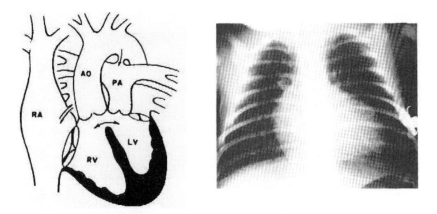

FIGURE 7-9. The transposition of the great vessels.

## Coarctation of Aorta

### *LOCATION*

The most common site is immediately beyond the origin of the subclavian artery.

### *IMAGING FINDINGS*

The classic chest x-ray appearance is rib notching (Fig. 7-10).

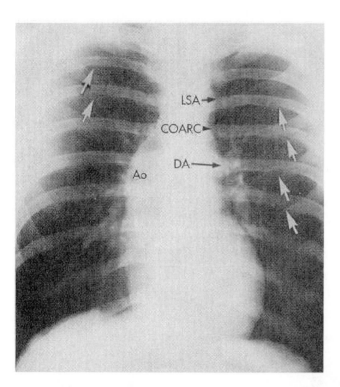

FIGURE 7-10. **Chest film from a patient with aortic coarctation, illustrating the components that contribute to the "figure-three" sign.**

HIGH-YIELD FACTS

Pediatric Radiology

Esophageal atresia is often associated with VACTERL anomalies.

- **V**—Vertebral anomalies
- **A**—Anal atresia (no hole at the bottom end of the intestine)
- **C**—Cardiac defect, most often ventricular septal defect
- **TE**—Tracheoesophageal fistula (communication between the esophagus and trachea) with esophageal atresia (part of the esophagus is not hollow)
- **R**—Renal (kidney) abnormalities
- **L**—Limb abnormalities, most often radial dysplasia (abnormal formation of the thumb or the radius bone in the forearm)

## Esophageal Atresia

### CAUSE

Blind-ending esophagus

### IMAGING FINDINGS

- Antenatal ultrasonography reveals polyhydramnios. However, diagnosis is usually made at birth.
- CXR may reveal air in blind upper end of esophagus (Fig. 7-11).
- Contrast studies with barium may reveal blind-ending esophagus with variable fistulous communication with the trachea (schematic).

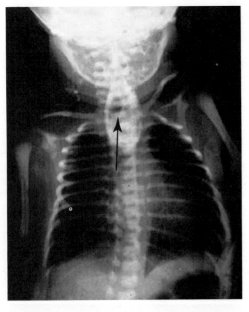
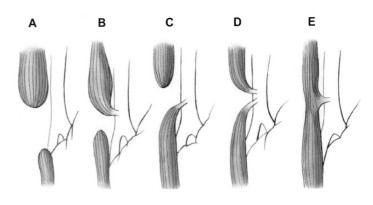

**FIGURE 7-11.** CXR demonstrating coiling of tube (arrow) secondary to tracheoesophageal (TE) fistula type C. The five types of TE fistulas (A–E) are labeled in the schematic.

240

*HIGH-YIELD FACTS*

*Pediatric Radiology*

## Pyloric Stenosis

### CAUSE

Genetic; more common in boys and Caucasians; occurs in 3 out of every 1000 births

### IMAGING FINDINGS

- Diagnosis confirmed by radiological testing using ultrasound or contrast studies.
- Ultrasound is extremely sensitive. Findings include elongated pyloric channel (> 14 mm) with thickened wall (> 4 mm).
- Radiographic signs on contrast studies include (Fig. 7-12):
  - String sign: Narrow, elongated pyloric channel
  - Shoulder sign: Pooling of barium in prepyloric antrum
  - Double tract sign: Nonspecific. Caused by two parallel barium streaks in the narrow pyloric channel.

Pyloric stenosis: Usually manifests at 4 weeks of age with progressive *nonbilious* vomiting after feeds. Most important physical finding is an "olive," which represents the thickened pylorus and can be palpated in the right upper quadrant.

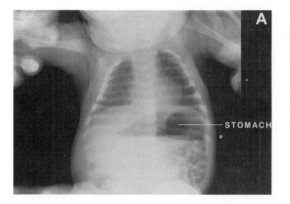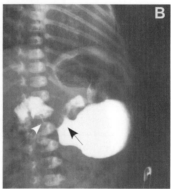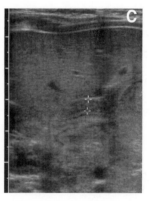

**FIGURE 7-12. Radiographic signs on contrast studies.**

Plate (A) is a plain abdominal radiograph depicting the "double bubble" sign in the stomach in a child with pyloric stenosis. Plate (B) is a barium study depicting the shoulder sign (black arrow) and the string sign (white arrow). Plate (C) is an ultrasound depicting thickened musculature (between calipers) in the pyloric region.

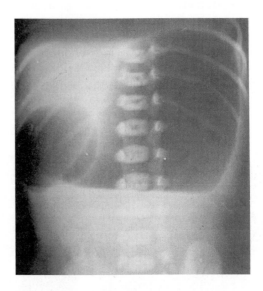

## Duodenal Atresia

**CAUSE**

Congenital

**IMAGING FINDINGS**

Diagnostic radiological sign on plain x-ray: "Double bubble" sign (Fig. 7-13)

> Duodenal atresia: Presentation at birth with *bilious* vomiting

**FIGURE 7-13. Duodenal atresia.**

Gas-filled and dilated stomach shows the classic "double bubble" appearance of duodenal atresia. Note that no distal gas is present. (Reproduced, with permission, from Rudolph CD, Rudolph AM, Hostetter MK, et al (eds): *Rudolph's Pediatrics*, 21st ed. New York: McGraw-Hill, 2003: 1403.)

## Volvulus

### CAUSE

Twisting of the intestine. May occur at the level of stomach as well

### IMAGING FINDINGS

- Diagnosis is confirmed by plain radiography or contrast studies.
- Plain x-ray may reveal obstruction with air fluid levels (Fig. 7-14).

Volvulus occurs in 1 in 500 live births in the United States.

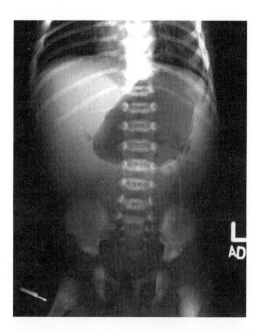

**FIGURE 7-14. Abdominal x-ray of a 10-day-old infant with bilious emesis.**

Note the dilated proximal bowel and the paucity of distal bowel gas, characteristic of a volvulus. (Reproduced, with permission, from Brunicardi FC, Andersen DK, Billiar TR, et al: *Schwartz's Principles of Surgery*, 8th ed. New York: McGraw-Hill, 2005: 1489.)

- Intussusception can be of different kinds, depending on the part of bowel involved: Ileoileal, ileocolic, colocolic
- The most common cause of intestinal obstruction in children

**Classic triad of intussusception:**
- Abdominal pain
- Vomiting
- Red currant jelly stools
- Seen in 21% of patients

### Intussusception

#### CAUSE

Sliding of a bowel loop into its distal portion.

#### IMAGING FINDINGS

- Plain x-ray provides indirect evidence of diagnosis. May be normal. Other findings include obstructive pattern, absence of intestinal gas in right lower quadrant, and free intraperitoneal air in severe cases with perforation.
- Ultrasound is a quick, noninvasive approach. Diagnostic features include swirled and "loop within loop" appearance of bowel loop ("target" or "donut" sign).
- Barium enema may be helpful in reduction in absence of peritoneal signs. May demonstrate the classic "claw sign" or coiled spring appearance caused by mucosal edema (Fig. 7-15).

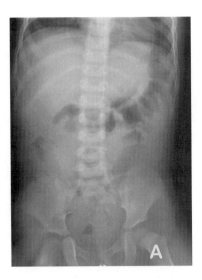
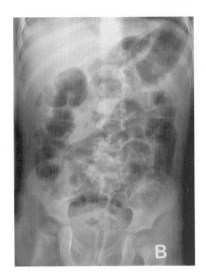
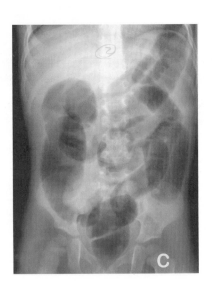

**FIGURE 7-15. Intussusception.**

Note the paucity of bowel gas in film (A). Air enema partially reduces it in film (B) and then completely reduces it in film (C). (Reproduced, with permission, from Stead LG, Stead SM, Kaufman MS: *First Aid for the Pediatrics Clerkship.* New York: McGraw-Hill, 2004: 132.)

## Necrotizing Enterocolitis

### CAUSE

Multifactorial. It is a result of inflammation or injury to the bowel wall secondary to infection or hypoxemia. More common in premature infants.

### IMAGING FINDINGS

- Scarce intraluminal gas
- Air within bowel wall (pneumatosis intestinalis) (Fig. 7-16)
- Free intraperitoneal air
- May also see gas within the portal system

Necrotizing enterocolitis is a surgical emergency in neonates.

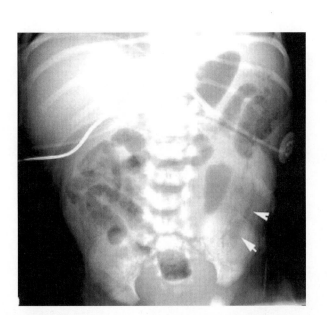

**FIGURE 7-16. Abdominal radiograph of infant with necrotizing enterocolitis.**

Note the presence of pneumatosis intestinalis (arrows). (Reproduced, with permission, from Brunicardi FC, Andersen DK, Billiar TR, et al. *Schwartz's Principles of Surgery*, 8th ed. New York: McGraw-Hill, 2005: 1493.)

### Cystic Diseases

#### CAUSE

Can be seen alone or in association with syndromes such as polycystic kidney disease, the infantile form of which is autosomal dominant

#### IMAGING FINDINGS

Diagnosis may be antenatal or postnatal on ultrasonography, which reveals enlarged hyperechoic kidneys (Fig. 7-17).

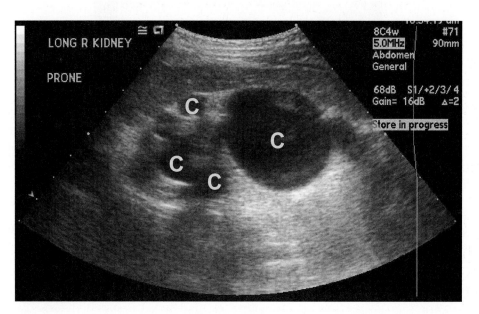

**FIGURE 7-17. Ultrasound demonstrating multiple hypoechoic cysts of various sizes in a child with multicystic kidney disease.**

## Renal Agenesis

### *IMAGING FINDINGS*

Presents as oligohydramnios on antenatal ultrasonography

## Wilms' Tumor

- Most common renal tumor in children
- Radiological diagnosis may be established by US or CT scan. Definitive diagnosis is histological (Fig. 7-18).

Renal agenesis may be unilateral or bilateral. Bilateral renal agenesis is incompatible with life.

Potter's syndrome is bilateral renal agenesis with pulmonary hypoplasia.

Wilms' tumor needs to be differentiated from neuroblastoma, which is extrarenal.

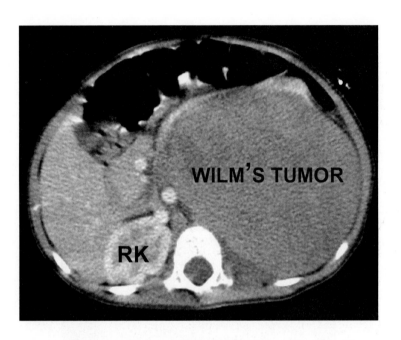

**FIGURE 7-18. Abdominal CT in a 3-year-old depicting a large left-sided Wilms' tumor (nephroblastoma) displacing adjoining vascular structures.**

# Horseshoe Kidney

### CAUSES

- Fusion of lower poles of bilateral kidneys
- Congenital

### IMAGING FINDINGS

- Intravenous pyelogram is often times diagnostic (Fig. 7-19).
- Findings are: malrotation, medial alignment of lower pole calyces, associated ureteropelvic junction obstruction.

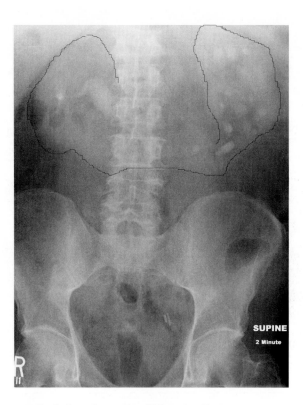

**FIGURE 7-19. KUB depicting a horseshoe kidney (outline).**

## Vesicoureteric Reflux

### CAUSES

- Abnormal retrograde flow of urine from the bladder into the ureters and kidneys.
- Most common causes are UTI, bladder outlet obstruction, detrusor instability, or congenitally short ureters.

### IMAGING FINDINGS

- Radiological approach: Voiding cystourethrogram (VCUG) and radionuclide cystograms (see Chapter 4).
- Ultrasound may reveal hydronephrosis and hydroureters (Fig. 7-20).

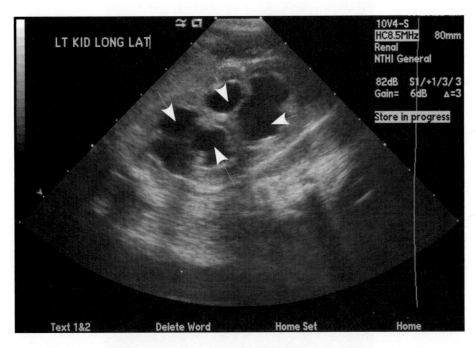

**FIGURE 7-20. Ultrasound demonstrating right hydronephrosis (arrows) in a newborn.**

### Posterior Urethral Valves

***CAUSE***

Congenital, occurs in males.

***IMAGING FINDINGS***

- Diagnosis is usually antenatal. Ultrasound reveals bilateral hydronephrosis in fetal kidneys and oligohydramnios.
- Male children with hydronephrosis on antenatal ultrasound should undergo voiding cystourethrogram (VCUG) soon after birth. It can reveal the dilated posterior urethra, up to the urethral valve, with bladder trabeculae, and in some cases vesicoureteric reflux (Fig. 7-21).

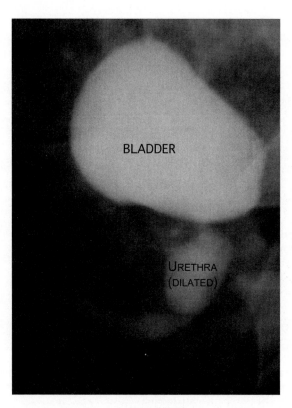

**FIGURE 7-21. Voiding (micturating) cystourethrogram showing dilated posterior urethra in a child with posterior urethral valves.**

## Scurvy

### CAUSE

Vitamin C deficiency. Usually dietary.

### LOCATION

Affects flat and long bones

### IMAGING FINDINGS (FIG. 7-22)

- Wimberger sign: Presence of a sclerotic rim around epiphysis
- White line of Frankel: Dense zone of provisional calcification at the growing metaphysis
- Trummerfield zone: A lucent zone below white line due to lack of mineralization
- Pelkan spurs: The area is prone to fractures manifesting at cortical margin
- Osteoporosis
- Subperiosteal hemorrhage

- Manifestations of scurvy are rare before 6 months of age.
- Characterized by:
  - Bony pains
  - Delayed skeletal growth
  - Bleeding gums
  - Rashes
  - Fatigue and irritability

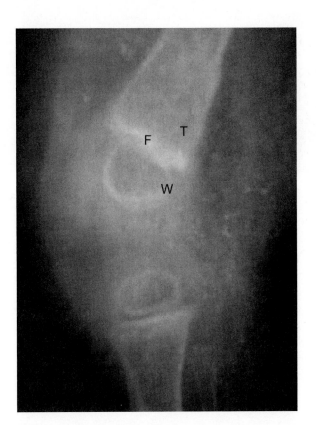

**FIGURE 7-22. Lateral view of knee joint depicting classical findings of scurvy. W, Wimberger sign; F, line of Frankel; and T, Trummerfield zone.**

HIGH-YIELD FACTS

Pediatric Radiology

Nutritional rickets is rare in the United States. Clinical manifestations:
- Muscular hypotonia
- Short stature
- Skull thickening

Knobby deformity in the chest—known as rachitic rosary

### Rickets

#### CAUSE

Vitamin D deficiency

#### IMAGING FINDINGS (FIG. 7-23)

- Plain radiography is diagnostic.
- Rickets can affect flat and tubular bones.
- Flat bones affected include skull and ribs.
- Typical findings in long tubular bones are noticed in the metaphyseal region (widening, cupping, and fraying due to lack of calcification of the osteoid).

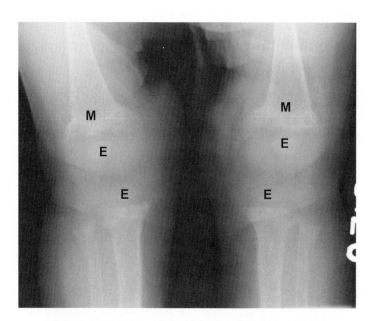

FIGURE 7-23. Lateral view of knee joint, depicting widening, cupping, and fraying of the metaphysis.

**Trauma—Long Bone Fractures and Salter-Harris Classification (Fig. 7-24)**

Salter-Harris Type I:
- Fracture through the physis (growth plate only)
- Often seen in children < 5 years
- Only visible radiographically if the physis is widened, distorted, or the epiphysis is distorted

Salter-Harris Type II:
- Through the metaphysis and the physis
- Most common sites are distal radius & tibia

Salter-Harris Type III:
- Through the epiphysis and physis
- Most common sites are knee and ankle

Salter-Harris Type IV:
- Through the epiphysis, physis, and metaphysis
- Most common site is lateral condyle of humerus
- Can produce joint deformity and chronic disability

Salter-Harris Type V:
- Crush injury of the physis
- May appear as a narrowing of the growth plate lucency
- Often not radiographically visible
- May lead to premature fusion
- The proximal tibia is the most common site for growth disturbance
- Mechanism is axial compression

**FIGURE 7-24. Salter-Harris classification.**

# Awards and Opportunities for Students Interested in Pursuing Radiology and Radiologic Specialties

### AMSER Henry Goldberg Medical Student Award

The AMSER Henry Goldberg Medical Student Award may be presented annually to any medical student who submits an outstanding abstract for a paper, poster, or electronic exhibit for presentation at the AUR Annual Meeting. Up to two awards may be presented annually. To be eligible, the work must have been performed while the applicant was a medical student. The candidate must be the first author or the presenter of the project.

The winning submission's author will receive a $500 honorarium and a certificate and will be acknowledged during the AUR Annual Meeting in the spring.

Submissions for the AMSER Henry Goldberg Medical Student Award competition cannot be simultaneously under consideration for award elsewhere.

To be considered for this award, an abstract MUST be submitted for presentation consideration at the AUR meeting and must be received by the abstract deadline.

### Association of University Radiologists (AUR) Memorial Award

In honor of deceased members of the Association of University Radiologists (AUR), a Memorial Award may be presented annually to the radiology medical student, resident or first year fellow who submits an outstanding original paper on any aspect of radiology. Eligible medical students, residents, or fellows may submit as the sole author of their paper, or they may do so in conjunction with other medical students, residents, or fellows and/or faculty. In the latter case, the medical student, resident or fellow must fully qualify as the senior author of the paper. **Only AUR members are eligible for this award.**

The winning paper will be published in Academic Radiology, and the author will receive a $1,000 honorarium, crystal award and certificate, and will be asked to present his or her essay during the AUR Annual Meeting. Note: All papers submitted for the award will be forwarded to the journal office of Academic Radiology for possible publication.

Manuscripts submitted for the Memorial Award Competition must be a first-time submission, cannot be simultaneously under consideration for publication or award elsewhere, and cannot be scheduled for presentation before the 2008 AUR Annual Meeting. Papers should not exceed 5,000 words and 10 illustrations, and tables must be kept within reasonable bounds. Otherwise, manuscripts should conform in all respects to the "Guidelines for Authors" found in Academic Radiology.

Deadline is in January. The winner will be notified in February.

For more information, contact the AUR Office by phone at 1-630-368-3730 or by email at AUR@rsna.org

CLASSIFIED

## Radiologic Society of North America (RSNA)
## Research Medical Student Grant

Eligibility:

- Full time medical student at accredited North American medical school.
- Project must take place in the department of radiology, radiation oncology, or nuclear medicine in a North American institution.
- $3,000 to be matched by sponsoring dept. Deadline: Year-round (Contact RSNA to check availability).

Radiological Society of North America (RSNA) www.rsna.org

RSNA Research and Education Foundation
820 Jorie Boulevard
Oak Brook, IL 60523
(630) 571-7816
(630) 571-7837 (FAX)
R&Efoundation@rsna.org

## Dr. Constantin Cope Medical Student Society for Interventional
## Radiology Annual Scientific Meeting Research Award

The purpose of the award is to introduce interested medical students to the greater interventional radiology community at the SIR Annual Scientific Meeting. The intent is to recognize the student author of an accepted abstract that best honors the spirit of inventiveness and scientific purity. Medical students in their second, third or fourth year at an accredited medical school who have demonstrated an interest in interventional radiology as a career and have participated in an original research project may apply.

The Annual Meeting Research Award Committee selects up to three recipients of this award each year.

Recipients will receive:

- Complimentary registration
- Travel award up to $1,000 payable toward the recipient's airfare, hotel and related meeting expenses
- Award recipient is responsible for any costs incurred beyond the total amount of the award. Read full reimbursement policy

Eligibility:

1. Primary Author must be a 2nd, 3rd or 4th year medical student at an accredited medical school, and must present the abstract as an oral presentation
2. Candidate need not be the principal investigator of the research project, but must have had a meaningful role in the research
3. Research must be original, and must have been conducted under the guidance of one or more SIR members, one of whom agrees to be present for the oral presentation

Required Materials:

1. Abstract Number; 2. Applicant's CV; 3. Letter of support from applicant's program director or department chair; 4. Letter of endorsement from an SIR member if the department chair or program director is not a member.

Abstract Submission Deadline: October; Applications due: November

All applicants will be notified of award status in early December. An applicant is only eligible to receive one research award from the SIR Foundation in any given academic year. For additional information, contact Jackie Cochran at awards@sirfoundation.org or phone (703) 691-1805.

## ▶ GENERAL MEDICAL STUDENT AWARDS

### AAMC Herbert W. Nickens Medical Student Scholarships

These awards consist of five scholarships given to outstanding students entering their third year of medical school who have shown leadership in efforts to eliminate inequities in medical education and health care and demonstrated leadership efforts in addressing educational, societal, and health care needs of minorities in the United States. Each recipient receives a $5,000 scholarship in November of the year the scholarships are awarded.

A medical school may nominate one student per year for this award. A candidate must be:

a U.S. citizen or permanent resident and

entering the third year of study in a LCME-accredited U.S. medical school in fall 2008. Students enrolled in combined degree programs (such as M.D./Ph.D.) are eligible when they are entering their third year of medical school.

a nomination letter from the medical school's dean or the dean's designate discussing the nominee's:

leadership efforts to eliminate inequities in medical education and health care,

demonstrated leadership efforts in addressing the educational, societal, and health-care needs of minorities,

excellent academic achievement through the first and second years of medical school (this is essential when a school has a pass/fail grading system),

awards and honors, special research projects, and extracurricular activities in which the student has shown leadership abilities;

a letter of recommendation from the medical school's designed minority affairs representative or office;

a letter of recommendation from a faculty member;

a personal statement by the nominee, which does not exceed 250 words, discussing his or her motivation for pursuing a medical career and how he or she anticipates working to improve the health and health care of minorities;

a curriculum vitae (CV) for the nominee which clearly indicates contact information; and

the nominee's official medical school academic transcript (remember to photocopy both sides of the transcript).

258

The deadline for receipt of nominations is in May. All nominations must be submitted to:

Herbert W. Nickens Medical Student Scholarships Award Committee c/o Juan Amador Association of American Medical Colleges, 2450 N Street, N.W., Washington, DC 20037-1127. For more information email nickensawards@aamc.org

## AAMC Caring for Community Grant Program

A National Medical Student Service Project Sponsored by the Pfizer Medical Humanities Initiative

Compassion and service are essential components of being a doctor. The increasing involvement of medical students in community service efforts demonstrates that they share this belief. The AAMC, with the support of the Pfizer Medical Humanities Initiative, is pleased to conduct an institutional grant program to encourage the development of student-initiated services and programs to the community. The AAMC manages a community service fund, the Caring for Community Grant Program, a philanthropy established to assist medical students who espouse and act upon their professional responsibilities to the community.

As part of the Caring for Community Grant Program, allopathic and osteopathic medical schools conferring the MD or DO degree are eligible to receive support for community service-oriented projects in which they explore new ways to serve their local communities. Eligible programs may range from those that promote awareness about sexually transmitted diseases, to vaccination and literacy programs, to any program that fulfills an unmet need within the community. Grant awards will also be offered to eligible service programs that are currently underway.

The unique aspect of the Caring for Community Grant Program is its focus on projects initiated, developed, and run primarily by medical students. While faculty and institutional involvement is integral to sustaining community service efforts, the ultimate goal of the Caring for Community Grant Program is to encourage students to identify untapped avenues of community service. Caring for Community will also help students to translate great ideas into meaningful service by contributing needed start-up and supplemental funds.

Applications will be processed and reviewed in March/April. Applicants will be notified of status by June.

For additional information, please contact:

Ally Anderson
Manager, Student and Community Service Programs
Association of American Medical Colleges
2450 N Street, NW
Washington, DC 20037
aanderson@aamc.org
202-828-0682

## Alpha Omega Alpha Medical Student Service Project Award

Purpose: To aid the establishment or expansion of a medical student service project benefiting the medical school or the local community, and to recognize students who dedicate their time and effort to these endeavors. Only one proposal will be accepted from a school during an academic year.

Eligibility: Any medical student or group of students at a school with an active AΩA chapter. AΩA membership is not required.

The award: The school will receive up to $2,000 per year, renewable for a second year up to $1,000 and a third year up to $500 to fund the project. Funding for the second and third years will be dependent on review by the national office of a progress report on the first year.

Dates: Applications will be accepted by the national office at any time.

Send applications to:

Medical Student Service Project Award
Alpha Omega Alpha
525 Middlefield Road, Suite 130
Menlo Park, California 94025

More information: Contact Ann Hill, (650) 329-0291,
a.hill@alphaomegaalpha.org

## American Medical Association Foundation Awards

The AMA Foundation will send a detailed packet of scholarship information to each medical school's Office of the Dean, Office of Student Affairs and Office of Financial Aid. It is through one of these offices that you can receive nomination and application information. It is the Office of the Dean or the Dean's Designate that must submit nominations to the AMA Foundation for the scholarships.

### PHYSICIANS OF TOMORROW SCHOLARSHIPS

These $10,000 scholarships reward current third-year medical students, who are entering their fourth-year of study. The selection of the recipients will be based on academic achievement and financial need.

There will be eight Physicians of Tomorrow scholarships funded by the AMA Foundation.

- The recipient of the one Physicians of Tomorrow Scholarship funded by the Audio-Digest Foundation should have an interest in "the communication of science." Activities such as mentoring and/or teaching are examples of "communication of science."
- The recipient of the one Physicians of Tomorrow Scholarship funded by the Johnson F. Hammond, MD Fund should have an interest in and commitment to a career in medical journalism.
- The recipient of the one Physicians of Tomorrow Scholarship funded by the Rock Sleyster, MD, Fund should have an interest in and commitment to a career in psychiatry.

260

Each medical school may submit one nomination for each of these scholarship opportunities. Thus, each school may submit up to four nominations in total.

Applications available: February 2008
Nominations due: May 30, 2008
Recipients announced:  August 2008

## MINORITY SCHOLARS AWARD

In collaboration with the Minority Affairs Consortium (MAC), with support from the Pfizer Medical Humanities Initiativeten Minority Scholars Awards are awarded annually, each in the amount of a $10,000 scholarship. You must be a current first- or second-year student and a permanent resident or citizen of the U.S. Eligible students of minority background include African American/Black, American Indian, Native Hawaiian, Alaska Native and Hispanic/Latino. Each medical school is invited to submit up to two nominees.

**Arthur N. Wilson, MD, Scholarship**—One $5,000 scholarship is awarded to a medical student who grew up in Southeast Alaska . Students may apply directly to the Foundation for this scholarship opportunity.

If you have questions about these scholarship opportunities, please contact:

Dina Lindenberg
Program Officer
(312) 464-4193
dina.lindenberg@ama-assn.org

### ▶ WEBSITES & RESOURCES OF INTEREST

## Radiological Society of North America Resources for Medical Students

- FREE Membership in RSNA
- FREE Attendance at the RSNA Annual Meeting
- FREE Access to the RSNA journals, RADIOLOGY and RadioGraphics.
- InteractED—Internet-based CME (free to all Medical Student Members)

## http://www.rsna.org/education/launchpad/index.html

- Extensive radiology education portal page from the RSNA
- Offers links for education in anatomy, radiology teaching files, health policy, medical ethics, physics, research, telemedicine, veterinary radiology and much more

## http://www.snm.org

- Educational page sponsored by the Society of Nuclear Medicine
- Five total online teaching files: pulmonary (1), bone (2), endocrine (2) —cases are presented in an Aunt Minnie style with stepwise introduction and teaching in the case with the opportunity for self-assessment (questions) throughout the discussion
- In-depth case discussion, mostly resident level

## http://learningradiology.com

- This is a fantastic website with lectures, pictures, and cases that teach radiology from the very beginning
- It is linked to a printed textbook, written by this website's author called Learning Radiology: Recognizing the Basics (Elsevier/Mosby) which uses the same fundamental approach to teaching as does this site, but contains key information on other modalities, additional material not covered on the website and access to StudentConsult.com with 50 interactive tutorials based on the book, including 240 imaged-based cases related to material in the book.

## http://radiologyweb.com

- This easy to navigate website features several interesting features including case of the month, resident's corner, CME/meetings finder, daily news and coding tips.
- A unique feature is its Asia Focus, which features leading articles by Asian radiologists, highlights radiology opportunities in Asia, and provides full text access to the Asian Oceanian Journal of Radiology.

## http://www.rsna.org/education/etoc.html#pulldowns

- Educational page sponsored by the Radiological Society of North America—offers interactive education, online journals and CME articles
- You must either be a member of the RSNA or pay fee to use these materials, in addition to registering with the site

## http://www.sbu.ac.uk/~dirt/museum/topics.html

- Educational radiology website from Central Middlesex Hospital (London)
- Tutorial for reading CXRs include viewing strategies, list of anatomical features, discussion on lung structure and function, etc.
- Text-based discussion with thumbnail images interspersed to illustrate points
- Introductory tutorial on basics of ultrasound

## http://www.radiology.wisc.edu/Med_Students/neuroradiology/NeuroRad/NeuroRad.htm

- Good tutorial for neuroradiology including neuroanatomy, vascular anatomy, neurofunctional systems, MRI & CT.
- Contains video files run through Windows Media Player that goes through anatomical images.

## http://www.med.wayne.edu/diagRadiology/Anatomy_Modules/Page1.html

- Radiographically based anatomy modules for brain, upper abdomen, thorax and pelvis-anatomy is taught from plain films and CT along with text-based explanations

## http://www.rad.washington.edu

- MSK anatomy tutorials taught from radiographs
- Mostly text-based with images throughout to illustrate points
- Quicktime movies on extremity CT/MRI

**http://everest.radiology.uiowa.edu/nlm/app/livertoc/liver/liver.html**

- University of Iowa website through department of surgery for learning the segmental anatomy of the liver
- Text-based discussion with thumbnail images and some Quicktime movies to demonstrate the segmental anatomy in three dimensions
- Approach is primarily a surgical vs. radiographic standpoint
- Mostly resident level

**http://www.ob-ultrasound.net**

- Tutorial webpage providing comprehensive review of the basics of OB ultrasound
- Linked to many different pictures, images, and teaching files of different diseases, equipment, anatomy and basic ultrasound physics

**http://www.radiology.co.uk/srs-x/tutorials.htm**

- Scottish Radiological Society educational resource page
- Provides text-based tutorials for lobar collapse, head CT in trauma and renal transplant
- Concepts are explained well with diagrams, tutorials are noninteractive

**http://www.mritutor.org/mritutor**

- Great basic tutorial in the basics of MRI
- One of the few tutorials on MRI
- Covers instrumentations, pulse sequences, artifacts, safety, contrast and more

# INDEX